All
Bagged
Up

With Love
Grahame
Howard
x

All
Bagged
Up

Grahame Howard

PNEUMA SPRINGS PUBLISHING UK

First Published 2009
Published by Pneuma Springs Publishing

All Bagged Up
Copyright © 2009   Grahame Howard
ISBN: 978-1-905809-47-9

Cover design, editing and typesetting by:
Pneuma Springs Publishing

A Subsidiary of Pneuma Springs Ltd.
7 Groveherst Road, Dartford Kent, DA1 5JD.
E: admin@pneumasprings.co.uk
W: www.pneumasprings.co.uk

A catalogue record for this book is available from the British Library.

Grahame Howard

INTRODUCTION

As a sufferer of Ulcerative Colitis for 10 years, Grahame Howard is well qualified to write about the humiliation and distress that this disease causes individuals on a daily basis.

Autobiographical in style, the book is written with the intention of reaching people with bowel disorders in such a way that they can relate to what they read helping them to realise that there are people who understand how they feel.

Ulcerative Colitis is described in detail, together with its possible causes, the medication used and its side effects. The book shows how the author lived and coped with the illness prior to major surgery for an ileostomy.

From thereon the emphasis is switched on to colostomy and ileostomy operations. Grahame Howard shows how he copes with the news that surgery is required and how he gradually learns to accept this news with many of the psychological battles and arguments occurring before being able to face up to the facts. There is also a section on people who have to undergo this type of surgery following an accident without receiving any prior warning.

Grahame's social work background comes into play as he deals with the issues of transition. He uses his coping skills and learns to accept the situation by facing the dilemma head on.

Heavily referenced with scripture references, together with explicit details of colostomy and ileostomy issues, Grahame explains in detail, the pros and cons of such a lifestyle with the intention of helping fellow sufferers realise that whatever has happened there is life out there for the taking. He takes the reader through such matters as changing appliances, what to look out for and ideas to help benefit them in their new life.

Throughout the book, the author's Christian faith shines through and he quotes many scriptures in an attempt to help the reader grasp how important and vital his faith in God is for his survival. He also shows how God performed a miracle in the hospital, helping him pull through the process of surgery.

Tension, frustration, anger and pain are all featured, as the author attempts to provide the reader with an honest but encouraging account of the life of an ileostomist.

CONTENTS

Grahame Howard

PREFACE

When I knew I would have to undergo stoma surgery, I set out to find more about what this entailed. Unfortunately I found the information somewhat limited. Apart from booklets about Ulcerative Colitis (UC) and colostomy and ileostomy surgery, there didn't appear to be anything written about the emotional trauma of coping with the drastic change in circumstances. There was also nothing about how ostomists, that is, those who have had either an ileostomy or a colostomy, managed their day-to-day lives living with a stoma, the artificial opening leading to the intestine.

I therefore decided to write my own account of how I managed as a UC sufferer for ten years, and how my Christian faith was very important in helping me face up to the reality of having a permanent ileostomy. Although initially difficult to manage, I found that once I had recovered from the operation the stoma immensely improved the quality of my life.

My main intention in writing this book is to assure anyone facing an ileostomy or colostomy that there is life after stoma surgery.

There are a few words used frequently throughout the text that need to be clearly understood. I explain them below.

Colectomy

A colectomy is the surgical removal of the entire colon, otherwise known as the large intestine. If only part of the colon is removed, the procedure is called a hemicolectomy. Following the removal, there may be a need, at least temporarily, for an opening to the intestine through the wall of the abdomen. Intestinal contents drain from this opening into a sealed pouch, a bag. The opening is known as a stoma, formed to replace the anus, and two types of operation to create a stoma may be performed, either a colostomy or an ileostomy. A proctocolectomy is an operation where part of the rectum and colon are removed and a panproctocolectomy, which is what I had, is where the entire rectum and colon are removed. The latter operation requires either a permanent opening of the ileum, the name for the last section of the small intestine, or the construction of an ileal pouch.

Colostomy

The word colostomy derives from the words 'colon' and 'stoma'. It is a surgical operation in which part of the colon is brought through the abdominal wall and opened to drain or decompress the intestine. The operation is designed to help the digestive system work normally, thus bypassing any damaged or inflamed area within the bowel. The colostomy may be temporary, eventually being closed to restore continuity, or permanent, usually when the rectum or lower colon has been removed. Surgery is used to divert waste into a stoma bag that is usually placed on the left-hand side of the abdomen, the part of the body that contains the digestive organs (better known as the belly), just below the belt line.

Ileostomy

The word ileostomy derives from the words 'ileum' and 'stoma'. An ileostomy is formed when the open end of the healthy ileum is diverted to the surface of the abdomen and secured there to form a new exit for waste matter as a stoma. This is usually on the right hand side of the abdomen, just below the belt line. An ileostomy is performed when waste matter has to be diverted away from part of the colon or rectum. This diversion is usually permanent if the large bowel and rectum are removed. There are, however, some occasions when a temporary ileostomy may be formed.

A colostomy operation may possibly be carried out by keyhole surgery, where only a very small incision is required and where the surgeon would be guided by a monitor screen for accuracy. Even if part of the colon had to be removed, it would not be nearly so serious an operation as an ileostomy.

With a permanent ileostomy keyhole surgery cannot be used. To remove the complete colon and rectum, the surgeon would need to make about a nine-inch incision. This operation is not reversible. There is a long recovery period required and there are very important psychological implications to be considered. It is a very major operation.

Ileo-anal pouch

With this operation, the diseased bowel and all or part of the rectum is removed but the sphincter muscles and anus are left in place. A pouch is constructed from the ileum and attached to the anus, so that it is still possible to defecate through the anus, but the use of the toilet will be more frequent. There will be a need for a temporary ileostomy while the newly-formed pouch is healing, but the stoma will be in place for only a couple of months.

1

A SHOCK

'I really think the only way forward is surgery,' said Dr Derwent, my consultant. 'We've tried every medication I can think of to help you, but sadly nothing has. To provide you with a better quality of life and to give your rectum a rest, I think a referral to Mr Rogers, the surgeon, would be a positive move, so that he can perform a colostomy operation.'

There was total silence in the consulting room, as I, along with my wife Hazel, tried to take in what Dr Derwent had just said. To say we were shocked would be an understatement. We felt devastated. Devastation, panic and fear mingled with a touch of disbelief, all rolled into one.

We had never considered surgery as an option. I had always believed, as a Christian, that I had already been healed according to God's Word (1 Peter 2:24), and that all I needed to do was to await the full manifestation of His healing in my life. Christians believe that Jesus heals people physically with the presence of the Holy Spirit. I believed that through my faith I would receive His healing and was waiting for the miracle to happen. To be faced with information that appeared to conflict with my belief was extremely distressing.

Problems had started about ten years previously. After many months of pain, distress and tests, I had been diagnosed with ulcerative colitis (UC). This was an inflammatory bowel disease that meant I urgently, and sometimes frequently, had to get to a toilet. I also had abdominal pains and a risk of other health problems.

As early as 1966, aged 20, I had experienced an occasional pain in my abdomen and the need to dash to the toilet. It hadn't worried me at the time, however. There had been no sign of blood or diarrhoea; not that I noticed anyway, it was just an annoying inconvenience. At that time I was working as a tool-setter on a twelve-hour shift system in a very busy factory. I never really had the time to think about what was happening to me. Perhaps because I was living in the fast lane I missed an early diagnosis. The problem appeared to settle down and only occasionally bothered me.

For over twenty-five years I didn't really have any particular worries. There was the odd pain from time to time, but I put this down to wind. I still had no visible signs of the disease such as blood or mucus, and I didn't as yet have to make frequent visits to the toilet.

In September 1990, however, I started to experience very severe pains in my abdomen. The pain was so intense that at times I wanted to cry out. If I was at home I would pace up and down, holding my stomach with the hope that the pain would subside. Usually it didn't. If I was away from home I really didn't want to do this and attempted to put on a brave face when really all I wanted to do was to shout out in agony.

With the pain came the urgent need to get to a toilet. A short while after the abdominal pain I would have a bowel movement. If a toilet was unavailable I wouldn't be able to control the bowel movement and would suffer the indignity of soiling myself. If I was at home I would be able to get to the toilet, although the experience of pain followed very quickly by the urgent need to evacuate my bowel would be tinged with panic, anger and distress. Out in public, of course, what happened would be devastating and I would have to think very quickly about how I could get to either a toilet, or, better still, home.

Shortly afterwards I started losing blood from my anus. This was extremely worrying and I began to fear that I might have cancer. My fears were aggravated by the fact that my mother had died of bowel cancer. At first there was just blood on the toilet paper and I thought that it was probably piles or some similar, easily treatable, problem. Thinking like this helped to accentuate my denial and alleviate my fear. My own diagnosis was short lived, however, as I began to have long spells of diarrhoea that contained blood and mucus.

I had mixed feelings at this time. Hazel and I trusted God wholeheartedly. We believed that He helped us to manage our lives and was our resting place. He kept us going through the confusion of the illness. He had the ability to heal me and to get rid of this disease, and I believed He would. Every time I had an accident I tried to keep my peace and hang on to my faith. Even though it was difficult, I found ways to praise and thank God. Not for what I was going through, but because I was better off than some people who had far worse to contend with.

I was only human, however, and this was noticeably apparent. I tried to pretend that there was nothing seriously wrong with me, but my fear became so intense that I finally agreed with Hazel that I should ask my doctor for advice.

At first the doctor was reluctant to make a diagnosis and suggested that I might have some type of 'bloodstained diarrhoea' or that it might be dysentery. After much insistence on my part, however, and a reminder that there was a history of bowel complaints in my family, he referred me to the local hospital to see a bowel specialist.

This was the first of many appointments with Dr Derwent, a kind and most helpful man with thinning hair and the oldest pair of brown NHS glasses that I had ever seen. He checked me over, prodding my stomach, and asked me various questions about what had been happening with my bowel. He then gave me a sigmoidoscopy examination. The sigmoidoscope consisted of a rigid, narrow tube, about as thick as an index finger and around twenty-five centimetres long. (It is made of stainless steel for durability.) This was passed through my anus to inspect the lining of the back passage and lower colon. The sigmoidoscope contained light conducting fibres that allowed Dr Derwent to examine the interior of the lower rectum and colon. It also contained a cutting tool so that he could take a biopsy. The procedure was not painful though it was quite uncomfortable, and as the sigmoidoscope passed through my anus it gave me the feeling that I was filled with air and that I would pass the contents of my bowel. I needn't have worried, however, because this didn't happen. (Even if it had, it wouldn't have mattered as the staff were used to dealing with such problems. They reassured me every inch of the way.)

With the test over, Dr Derwent was able to confirm that I had UC and that it was quite 'angry'. I had mixed emotions. I was relieved that it was UC and not bowel cancer, but was scared about the future and how I would cope with ill health. I was also at a loss to know why God had allowed my ill health to exist. Hazel and I had, to the best of our knowledge, been faithful to God and believed in everything the Bible said. Why then was this happening? Why was I not being healed? I had many questions that needed answers.

I decided as a starting point that I would research UC, as from now on the disease would clearly be part of my everyday existence. I found that UC is a debilitating disease, in which the lining of the colon and rectum become severely inflamed and may eventually wear away forming sores known as ulcers. The colon is often permanently damaged. It is an ongoing or chronic condition and produces symptoms that come and go, even when treated. The disease is unpredictable: following a relapse it can go into remission.

Although the disease can occur at any age, signs of it tend to show in early adolescence. Most people with UC have inflammation in the section of the large intestine stretching from the left side of the abdomen to the pelvis, or in the sigmoid colon, the section of the intestine joined to the rectum. Others, however, may have inflammation throughout the whole of the intestine.

Most people have only mild or moderate forms of the disease. Symptoms may include rectal bleeding, diarrhoea and mucus. All these symptoms can be controlled by medication. Others may have a more severe form of the disease, with extensive bouts of diarrhoea, stomach pain and fever. When this happens, the inflamed colon is unable to function properly in removing water from the stools. Diarrhoea may be frequent, both day and night. Other problems may include arthritis, liver problems and leg ulcers. In addition, patients who have had UC affecting the entire colon for ten or more years have a major risk of cancer.

Why UC occurs is as yet unknown, in spite of over forty years of research into the disease. There are a number of possible causes. For example, it is suggested that stress may worsen the symptoms of colitis. I know from my own experience that when I become anxious or upset about anything, I risk a bad attack of colitis. When my brother died suddenly, for instance, the grief, anxiety and shock led to a major attack. I think it's very possible that stress promotes an attack.

It is thought that certain foods and drinks can affect or trigger the symptoms of UC in some people. There is, however, no ideal diet for sufferers. Something that is eaten and aggravates one person may be perfectly all right for someone else. One man's meat may certainly be another man's poison. Unfortunately, as I found out, diet is a case of trial and error. For instance, I was told to avoid dairy products as they might trigger an attack, but found there was no substance to this statement at all and have continued to enjoy these foods. Obviously it is wise when having an attack of UC not to eat or drink certain foods that are known to aggravate diarrhoea. At such times foods that exacerbate the condition, for example, fruit, onions, beer and fatty foods, should be avoided. If you have stomach cramps caused by a narrowing of the intestine, you should also avoid foods that are hard to digest, such as dried fruits, nuts and gristle, as the pain may be increased.

Most scientists who specialise in IBD believe that some people have a genetic susceptibility to the condition. Evidence for this comes from the large number of children with UC with a close family member who also suffers from the disease. Genetic susceptibility is certainly relevant so far as I'm concerned. My mother not only suffered from bowel cancer but also from UC, and it is thought she died of bowel cancer because the UC was left untreated. She decided, possibly because of the embarrassing and also frightening symptoms, 'not to bother the doctor because he's busy enough', a statement she made frequently. Furthermore, my eldest daughter has suffered from UC for many years. She was diagnosed in 1980, ten years before I experienced major symptoms of the disease.

Research continues into UC, and I am sure that one day soon a more accurate assessment of the causes will be found. Until then, however, sufferers will have to learn to live with the disease and find ways that make life easier to cope with.

For the first few years following diagnosis, the disease in my body, although rampant at times, was controlled by medication. UC sufferers have to take medication every day for life. Even so, the disease may flare up and become extremely 'angry', and can then go into remission some months later. During the 'angry' stage, large doses of medication have to be taken to reduce inflammation.

Initially following diagnosis, the medication I was prescribed worked quite well. To start with, I was prescribed four 400 mg Mesalazine (Asacol) tablets a day. Mesalazine is an anti-inflammatory drug that helps to reduce inflammation in the rectum and colon. It also helps to prevent further episodes of UC. I also had to apply Predsol retention enemas rectally.

Predsol is a steroid drug that helps to dampen down inflammation localised in the rectum or colon. The enemas were applied daily whilst inflammation persisted. (One was usually applied before bedtime, but when I was really unwell I also had to have one in the morning as well as one in the evening.) Somewhat later I was prescribed 50 mg Azathioprine tablets twice daily. This particular medication also helps to reduce inflammation in UC. These drugs may control mild or moderate forms of UC. When the condition becomes more serious, however, strong anti-inflammatory drugs such as corticosteroids, for example Prednisolone, may be prescribed to help counter the inflammation. I took corticosteroids on a number of occasions, starting with a dose of 40 mg per day that consisted of eight 5 mg tablets taken in two doses of four tablets daily. I took this dose for two weeks and then took a reduced dose of six tablets daily for a fortnight, gradually reducing the dose until I had completed the course of treatment. Prednisolone tablets are very effective, but unfortunately the side effects can be daunting. These can include slow growth in children, indigestion, peptic ulcers, an increased appetite, weight gain, a swollen abdomen, ulceration and thrush of the throat. Side effects may also include unusual growth of body hair, fatigue or drowsiness, swollen feet or ankles, high blood pressure, muscle weakness, brittle bones, acne, thinning of the skin leading to bruising, broken veins, slow healing, mood swings and insomnia.

I suffered a number of these side effects. My face looked like a large apple as it ballooned in size. The correct term is 'moon-faced'. I also put on a lot of weight, and had to buy new clothes as I increased in girth. Sleeping was also a problem. I would often be up at 2 a.m. suffering from insomnia. Mood swings often dominated my life at this time. Sometimes I would be quite happy, and then for no apparent reason would either be angry or down in the dumps.

In the early part of 1998, after eight years of continuous medication of varying sorts and bouts of flare-ups and remissions, the UC flared up again quite nastily. In June of that year I had to take time off sick from my job as a social worker with a local authority. I was off sick for six months, and with no sign of improvement in my health I then had to take ill health retirement.

This was devastating. I had worked very hard to achieve my position within the social services and had enjoyed the work immensely. With good prospects ahead, I had been looking forward to a long and successful career. This was not to be, however, and I felt very downcast and rejected. I was suffering loss: loss of good health and loss of a good career. The losses were to bring great changes into my life. Not many people really like change, and I felt that changes were being forced upon me in a very cruel way that I couldn't control. They were changes that I had never thought would happen.

In December 1998 I retired from my position as a social worker and was reduced to drawing incapacity benefit. This was quite a shock as I had been used to a good salary. I was now learning what it was like to be on a much lower income.

Having left the social services, I was given a lump sum as well as a monthly pension. With careful planning, I worked out that I could make the lump sum last for about eighteen months and still live comfortably. I adjusted quite well into my new life. Unfortunately, however, as soon as I took a step forward, the disease pushed me back much further than any steps taken forward.

Most adults need to visit the toilet perhaps three or four times a day. A UC sufferer quite often loses count of the many times he or she needs to 'go'. I needed to go on average between twelve to fifteen times every day, sometimes more, and was often in dreadful pain. Furthermore, the unpredictability of the disease was catching me unawares. Many times whilst I was out shopping or taking the dog for a walk I suffered the indignity of having an 'accident' right where I was.

21

No one knows better than a sufferer just how urgent urgent can be. Before you know it, disaster has struck, and you are left wondering just how you are going to get home and what you should do.

Problems loom large in a UC sufferer's mind. If you are going to manage, you have to use your mind. If you are not mentally in charge of what is going on, for instance, you might not want to go out at all, fearing that you might need to go to the toilet and get caught out. I know this from experience and I really had to think hard to stop being too upset to go out at all or to do anything.

To deal with the UC, which meant wanting to evacuate my bowl suddenly, very fast and without any warning, I began taking emergency packs with me whenever I could. These would contain wet wipes, toilet paper, clean underwear, a disposable bag and medication. There were limitations as to where I could take these items, but usually I took them if I was going out in the car. Even then, I would find out where the nearest toilets were and plan how to get to them, just in case.

Walks were worrying, and I had many accidents when I thought I would be all right but unfortunately was caught short. Suddenly along the route, and without warning, I would need to have a bowel movement. All attempts to control this were impossible, and I was left stranded and extremely distressed.

The washing machine was on the go practically all day, as my wife Hazel faithfully tried to keep up with the constant demand of dirty washing. Many times I told her to leave the clothes for me to deal with. Sometimes, frustrated beyond endurance, I would throw them away. Nevertheless, Hazel understood my frustration and what I was going through, and didn't let me down. I am so grateful to her and to God for giving her to me.

I must be honest: there were times when I felt she deserved

better and suggested she would be better off finding someone else. She just shrugged my suggestion aside, however, and refused to stop loving me.

I felt angry and sad. Yet within me, I couldn't forget that eighteen years earlier I had become a Christian by giving my life to Jesus. No matter what I was going through, it would be nothing in comparison to what Jesus suffered for me. As a Christian, I believed that Jesus hung in brutal agony on a cross for the sins of the world. He did not deserve the pain or to be treated in such a barbaric manner. Yet he didn't complain or fight back. He just received the pain for all who would believe in Him, and who thus received forgiveness of their sins and eternal life. Though I hurt, and felt beaten and deserted, as I focused on the one thing that had kept me going during all those years, I could not fail to give God the glory.

It was only the beginning, and there would be many days when I would not feel like praising God or thanking him. My faith would be tested to the limit.

2

TENSIONS MOUNT

We left the specialist's consulting room in silence. There was a lot to think about before we could go any further. Hazel and I were in shock. We needed to come to terms with what had been said before we could begin to make any sense of the situation.

'Why me?' figured strongly in my thinking. Hazel, who has always been the more reflective of the two of us, said little but tried to listen to my reasoning.

'We'll get through this,' she said to me. 'We really will.' But I knew she was saying this only to keep me going. Deep down, I could tell she was as worried as I was about what was going to happen.

We both found talking to each other very therapeutic. We sat for hours bouncing ideas off each other. What we didn't know about UC we found from books or the Internet. I am a little sceptical about information to be found on the Internet, so I tried to stick to reliable sites such as The National Association for Colitis and Crohn's (NACC), The British Colostomy Association and other health information services. (The addresses for these, along with other reliable institutions, can be found at the end of the book in the 'Useful Information' section on page 151.

Spending time with each other and attempting to reassure

ourselves that whatever might happen would work out brought us great release. The information we needed and found helped us to have the confidence to face family and friends with the news of what was going to happen.

During the next few weeks we began to gather further information about colostomy operations and talk through the situation with family and close friends. It is not easy to tell people you have to have stoma surgery, and, to be blunt, to make it clear to people who have no knowledge of UC that you're going to have a bag attached to your abdomen for the rest of your life. Whether friends or family, the subject is still very embarrassing, and you can never be sure of how anyone will react. What is certain is that the subject is a conversation stopper.

As my savings were running out, I took myself off incapacity benefit and began to work on a self-employed basis as a pastoral social worker for my church. This was only for two mornings a week, but it helped: it provided money, vital for our standard of living, and also boosted my pension. The job was also therapeutic from an emotional point of view.

My GP was at first reluctant to let me work again, but he finally agreed to this as long as I didn't overdo things. In fact, the job worked well because not many people attended church during the day, and I had easy access to a toilet. It also gave Hazel a well-earned break for two mornings a week.

The UC was now wrecking my body and was causing both Hazel and myself much misery. I would often say 'I can't take much more of this. I'd be better off dead.'

In retrospect I know this was a selfish statement to make, but one over which I had no control. I was very depressed. I was very anxious and couldn't cope with anything. It was the loss and change that I was finding hard to accept and adjust to. I had a fear of the unknown and because I couldn't think of the future in any clear way at all, everything became frustrating.

The information we had gathered helped, but the unknown path forward was frightening to contemplate. The loss, change and dread of the future led to a great feeling of tiredness and lethargy that I found difficult to pull myself out of.

My GP prescribed some anti-depressants to help counteract the hopelessness and lethargy and to help me sleep better. Unfortunately, though, I had to stop taking the anti-depressants after a week as they not only relieved my anxiety but also relaxed my bowel and I began to experience great difficulty in passing a motion. I continually wanted to evacuate the waste, but my rectum refused to comply. This resulted in further bleeding and excruciating pain.

I began to feel a prisoner in my own home. I had previously been going to church every Sunday morning, but now had to stop attending as it was causing me distress. With about 150 males in the congregation, including children, and only one male toilet, going to church was a recipe for disaster and one from which I preferred to abstain.

I began to feel very sorry for myself and became even more irritable. Everything was now so frustrating when previously things had seemed so positive. My social work career had been forging ahead and up until 1998 the UC had been manageable to a degree helped by constant medication. Now my future seemed unbearably bleak. The sadness I felt was overwhelming.

I began to shout at Hazel. I began to shout at God. I blamed both of them for what had happened to me. I would snap at Hazel and then apologise, only to repeat the snapping within a very short space of time. I treated God the same way. In retrospect, I think the bad behaviour was caused by the way I was living and my method of trying to cope with the disease. It may also have been from the side effects of steroid treatment that can cause mood changes.

As a Christian I felt and behaved like a yoyo. One minute I

was up and for God, but the next moment I was down and blaming Him for my predicament. I still could not understand why God, whom I believed loved me enough to send His Son Jesus to die in my place on the cross, would not honour my faith and trust in Him and grant me healing. This confused and hurt me. I was faced with a dilemma as I had lived as a man of faith and had preached regularly on the subject. Now I wondered how I could preach healing to people when God hadn't healed me. It didn't seem to make sense.

I felt as though I was two people. One moment I was hanging on to all I knew as a Christian and trying to live my life as such. But the next moment I was in despair and couldn't see how I was going to cope with the necessary drastic changes required for the way I had to live in the future. Something needed to happen to help me manage my life that had become so very difficult. I struggled with the problem for a while.

Then one July afternoon, as I sat in the hot sunshine, I felt that God spoke to me. The substance of what He said was as follows:

> 'Grahame, My thoughts are not like your thoughts and My ways are very different to yours. At times it is difficult for people to know what I am doing or why a particular thing has happened. My word says you're healed. You and Hazel have remained focused on this, but up to now you have not received the manifestation of my healing. Fear not, this is My will. As a result of what has happened to you, I will open the way for you to help people in need. Don't try to work out how I will do this, because you will not be able to do so. I will show you later. Until then, know I am always with you and care about you. You will come through the operation and convalescence successfully. Don't worry about money, work, or how other things will be done. Just know they will be. You and Hazel have nothing to fear. I love you both dearly.'

As I reflected on what God had told me, I began to feel His love and His peace envelop me. This is not easy to put into words. I just knew He was there and that He knew how I felt. I felt a new faith within me.

I began to re-focus my thoughts and think things through more positively. It was not easy. I attempted to look at things more realistically and as obstacles flagged up in my mind, tried to visualise them as small and manageable problems. I began to focus on my goal to live life as normally as possible and then realised I could manage the problems. I remembered how the runner Linford Christie used to prepare himself for a race. He would make his eyes bulge out. This gave him tunnel vision, helping him to block out everything either side of him. He only had to concentrate on the way ahead. This was the impetus I needed and I decided to try to put my thoughts into practice.

Later, while I was studying the Bible, I felt God was showing me that there was a purpose to the pain that I was experiencing. He helped me to focus on the fact that only damaged people can re-build themselves; those who are whole have no need of repair.

I realised that God does not waste experience. All of us experience things that we never imagined could happen to us, and I was no exception.

I began to see that I could possibly help other people by writing down my thoughts. I knew what it was like to suffer from UC. I was now beginning to understand the emotional trauma of trying to come to terms with stoma surgery. Very soon I reckoned I would be able to write about everyday life with a stoma. I felt this might benefit other people in a similar situation.

There it was, loud and clear: a purpose. I had something to hang on to. A hope. I felt that the reason why I was going through all this suffering was to help reach my fellow sufferers who had no particular hope. The means of being able to reach them was to have experienced what they had gone or were going through. I was beginning to receive answers to my endless search for a meaning. I also began to see that if I could help others in letting them know how I had coped, these others might help yet others. The learning process could be passed along in a chain, bringing some peace of mind to many like myself who have suffered and have longed for release. (In the New Testament, Paul says that God helps us through the troubles and hardships that we find ourselves in, so that we in turn may be able to offer help to others who are living in troublesome times – 2 Corinthians 1:4.)

Now I felt I knew the reason why I had not been healed and the purpose for which I had been chosen. It was almost as if God was saying to me: 'Since you have known Me, you've professed to being a man of faith; let's see if you really are.'

It still seemed strange that God should choose to use me like this. I felt He was giving me a deeper insight into His ways and leading me into new things. I decided to continue to change my thinking in order to remain focused. In the past I had often met others who were going through a crisis in their lives and had said 'I know how you feel'. But I now realised that I couldn't know how they felt unless I myself had been through the same or very similar experience. How could I begin to understand what people were experiencing or how they were feeling unless I really knew myself?

Earlier, when things had not turned out the way I had expected them to, I had been left in much confusion and often sought for a reason why things happened the way they did. Sometimes if someone was not healed I was tempted to think there might be a sin in his or her life that was preventing the healing. I based my thinking on Psalm 66:18 which says 'If I regard iniquity in my heart, the Lord will not hear'. Christians believe that sin or wrongdoing blocks their way to God. Jesus came to mankind to set people free from the sin that separates them from Him. For a Christian, failure to receive an answer to a prayer may well mean there is something preventing the prayer reaching God. This might have been true, but also God might have been doing something leading to the fulfilment of His purpose.

Back in 1980 I asked the Lord Jesus into my life and told Him I would serve Him and do whatever He asked of me. I could hardly complain by thinking how unreasonable He was, having made such a commitment.

My Christian beliefs may conflict with those of other people. I write from experience and about what I believe in. I don't want to persuade the reader to accept everything I say as authoritative, but I do want to show that I did things my way and that, for me, my way works. Others may have different beliefs; if so, I respect them. My aim is to encourage the reader that, when times are hard, it is so useful to have something to believe in. It's a matter of what feels right and gives inner peace. I have found it so helpful to have a belief to hold on to when times are hard. My Christian faith has helped me through very difficult times, although there have been times when I've felt like giving it all up.

I now had a purpose and a goal to set my sights on. I was, however, still very scared, and was definitely not looking forward to going into hospital. I carried on each day, albeit with a struggle at times, and there were some days I woke up thinking that I couldn't bear another day.

I contacted social services to find out if they could assist with providing a second toilet in my house. I was spending a lot of time each day in the lavatory, and this was beginning to become a problem for friends and family who also wanted to use the little room occasionally. There were also problems if the toilet was engaged and I needed to get there urgently.

Having assessed my situation, social services came to the conclusion that I was a Priority 1 case, and that a second toilet would greatly improve the quality of my life. They set about putting the wheels in motion for assistance. In the interim they provided me with a commode. This was a great shock and at first I refused to consider using such a thing. Within a short time, however, I'd swallowed my pride and strategically placed the commode in our downstairs bathroom, which didn't have a toilet. I used it in emergencies – gratefully.

I applied for and was given a blue disabled parking badge, which was also gratefully accepted. Until then, I had often been out driving and had felt the urgent need to use a toilet, but because of yellow lines or nowhere to park had suffered an accident. The badge enabled me to park near a public convenience and saved me from distress and embarrassment.

Hazel says that I was more pleased with receiving the blue badge than I was with receiving my birthday presents. I have to confess that the day it arrived I went into town and refused to park anywhere except on yellow lines or in a disabled parking area. Unfortunately that day the town was extremely busy with traffic and I had to drive around the town for twenty minutes before I could find a space.

I found it difficult to come to terms with the fact that I myself was now a service user (client) rather than a social worker, but eventually realised this was something I had to accept and not let it become a major problem.

Reading the Bible one day, I was reminded that Christians are called upon to rejoice and be happy, and how important this is. For example, 'Rejoice in the Lord always. Again I will say, rejoice.' (Philippians 4:4), and 'Rejoice always' (Thessalonians 5:16). There is also 'Do not sorrow, for the joy of the Lord is your strength' (Nehemiah 8:10).

It is so easy to begin to feel sorry for yourself, to internalise everything and become embittered with problems. Scripture encourages us to rejoice in what happens to us, in other words, to laugh through life. Laughing is medicine for our souls: 'A merry heart does good, like medicine /But a broken spirit dries the bones.' (Proverbs 17:22).

Laughing really was not easy. It took a tremendous effort at times to praise the Lord and be joyful through the hard times. Also, to laugh my way through everything often stuck in my gullet. Nevertheless, laughter was vital. I tried very hard to laugh, focusing on the times when I had to give myself retention enemas and started to see the funny side of things.

There were occasions when Hazel and I laughed a lot at the antics and positions I needed to get into when trying to apply the enemas. They are steroid-based and housed in very soft, supple sachets, rather like hair gel. The idea is to insert the spout into the rectum and then roll the sachet up, thus forcing the liquid in. This is done by lying on your back or turning on to your side.

As I'm sure many sufferers will agree, however, the application is not always successful and I often had to improvise. Some days I had to hoist my legs up into the air from a lying position while I applied the liquid. My legs often touched the wall behind me until I was very nearly standing on my head. If I happened to look at Hazel at the time, we would both fall into silly giggles and I would collapse into a heap on the bed convulsed with laughter. It brought a wonderful release, and helped me to cope when thinking about the future.

One of the most embarrassing characteristics of being a UC sufferer is breaking wind in a very different way to most other people. Hazel and I would often laugh as I emitted very awesome and long-lasting sounds. Sometimes these would occur as I walked along, noisily pop-pop-popping. Hazel would often say 'I think you could play a tune with that,' and we would laugh hysterically. There was nothing else to do but laugh, and laughing made us both feel ever so much better.

I realised that if I did not rejoice, as God's word was

encouraging me to do, I would not be able to live. If I rejoiced, I would find the necessary strength to help me live through the situation I was in. It was my choice as to whether the glass was half empty or half full, that is, whether I saw my situation from a negative or positive standpoint. Much depended on the way I perceived things. I chose, at first with difficulty, to be positive in the way I thought about things.

Bitterness can spread within us like a cancer. I began to see that if I adopted a negative standpoint, it made me feel bitter. I saw how easy it was to blame other people for what I was going through. I also realised I could begin to dwell on the unfairness of my situation if I were not careful. This would be a pointless exercise.

I came to the conclusion that dwelling on the negative side of things was pointless unless I had some means to rectify the situation. I thought it far wiser to stop thinking negatively, difficult though this was, and to look positively at what could possibly be salvaged in what appeared to be a hopeless situation.

Rejoicing and learning to laugh at myself through whatever circumstance I found myself in brought such a release. It also helped me to see things more clearly and logically. I do stress this was not easy, but with practice I managed to rejoice and laugh.

I would very much need to remember to laugh and rejoice in the days ahead, as there was another shock in store.

3

Job's Comforters and a Further Shock

As a social worker and counsellor, I knew that my job was not to solve other people's problems by putting ideas into their heads or inflicting my opinions upon them. Rather, it was to help them find solutions to the predicaments they were in, thus promoting their cognitive skills and coping abilities. This would mean I would have to assess my clients' situations very carefully so that I knew and understood what was happening to them, and then by listening, showing them I am listening by using good attending skills and using eye contact, present certain options that might be able to help them through the troublesome circumstances they were in as well as build up their confidence.

Unfortunately, certain people I was in contact with when I first learnt of the need for my serious operation did not treat me like this. Some felt they needed to demonstrate their own problem-solving skills. I came across a number of well-meaning people who suddenly knew why I was ill and why I hadn't been healed. Some even discovered they were UC experts, and were certain what had caused it or triggered it off. A typical conversation would be as follows:

'How do you know it's colitis? It might be a bug.'

'I know it is,' I would reply, 'I've had it for years.'

'It could be what my aunt had,' the person would insist. 'She picked up something when she went to Spain on holiday. It lasted for months. It sounds just like what she had. Come to think of it, my stomach's not been too good either. I keep having to go to the loo.'

'It's nothing like that,' I would say, trying to defend myself. 'UC is a disease that needs constant medical treatment. There is a loss of blood and mucus.'

'I've had that as well,' would be the reply.

Even though it was only a few people who behaved like this, their talk made me feel very frustrated.

From a spiritual point of view, I began to realise how Job may have felt when his supposed friends came to visit him, only to conclude that his suffering was a direct result of his wicked sinfulness. Some of my visitors began to probe me to establish if there was any unconfessed sin in my life, or if I needed to forgive someone else, or was feeling bitterness against anyone.

'What have you been up to, then?' came one enquiry from someone who thought I should have been healed.

'What do you mean? I asked.

'Well, you must have been in sin or God would have healed you, wouldn't He?'

On another occasion, someone asked me whether there was something in my past.

'Why do you ask?' I said.

'What I mean,' the person continued, 'was that I wondered whether you were holding any resentment against anyone. Or perhaps you haven't forgiven someone for a wrongdoing. The sin may be blocking healing from God.'

Although it did help to look within myself to find out if they were right, I nevertheless found this a futile exercise.

Some attempted to water down the UC symptoms, suggesting

they were all in my mind. One person who claimed to have had a lot of experience with UC asked me whether I'd had any counselling.

'What for?' I replied.

'For the so-called attack of colitis that you've been complaining about. Counselling could help you see that it's all in the mind.'

'Do you mean that it's psychosomatic?' I retorted. 'Are you trying to tell me that I'm imagining all this?'

'Well, in a way you are,' came the reply. 'If you went to the clinic that my friend went to, the people there would help to train your mind. They would help you to understand that because of your nervousness and fear of having an accident, you are signalling to your rectum that you need to go to the loo. The people at the clinic would help you re-think things through.

With spastic or nervous colitis, a mild form of colitis, this may be true, but it's certainly not the case with UC. The former has indeed been described as psychosomatic in origin. It is usually a temporary upset rather than a chronic inflammation. Treatment of this disorder tends to be provided with psychological support. With UC, however, which has many adverse symptoms caused by inflammation, this is not the case.

I would have given anything to be able to train my mind to send signals to my rectum, specifying in no uncertain terms that I didn't have to go to the toilet. All UC sufferers know, however, that the disease is entirely unpredictable and that it is likely to strike at the most inopportune times. To be in control of my bowel movements would certainly have improved the quality of my life and would have allowed me to control an important part of my bodily functions. But UC can be cruel.

People can also be cruel. At a time when I needed

encouragement and understanding, I was instead sometimes subject to unhelpful contributions that I could well have done without.

'I've brought these Imodium for you to try,' said a visitor to the house. 'They'll soon clear up the runs and get you back on your feet.'

Someone else said,' You should watch what you eat. It's to do with diet, young man, mark my words.'

In fact, all I needed from the people I knew was tender loving care, love and understanding, and someone to talk to.

Hazel had no one with whom she could really share her concerns. There was her sister, but she lived in Cambridgeshire, far away from us. They often talked to each other on the phone, but she needed someone who would sit down and just listen to her worries.

Quite often we were with people who talked to us. That, however, was the problem. We needed people who would listen. Listening is a skill. It requires the ability to attend to someone, to show you are really listening and possibly provide a little feedback in the conversation. We may be tempted to listen a bit and then immediately offer lots of problem-solving tips, without really having taken in what the person we are talking to has been saying. People with major problems, however, often want someone who will be there just for them, without any preconceived ideas or solutions. Hazel was desperate for someone like that. Sadly, that someone was not there for her, or for me, either.

Nevertheless, I have to say that most people were helpful and supportive. Looking back, I don't think we could have managed without their love, prayers and support. Both Hazel and I are very grateful to them.

The day finally arrived when I was to see the surgeon. The appointment was not until 3 p.m. so I had plenty of time to prepare myself and calm my nerves.

I began the day reading a little scripture, and felt that God gave me a verse from Hebrews: 'The Lord is my helper, I will not fear. What can man do to me?' (Hebrews 13:6).

I felt greatly encouraged by this and later shared the verse with Hazel while we had a cup of coffee. When I said to her 'What can man do to me?' she replied jokingly, 'He can cut your belly open.'

For a split second there was silence. Then, as we realised what she had said, we fell about laughing. It brought a wonderful release from the pent up fear that was trying to engulf me. But little did we know just how much of my belly would need to be cut open.

'Well, Mr Howard,' Mr Rogers the surgeon began as he completed a sigmoidoscopy on me, 'it is quite angry in the rectum and the colonoscopy that you had two years ago showed your entire colon is affected by the colitis. When it gets this far, and bearing in mind you were diagnosed ten years ago, we certainly have to consider surgery. In this instance a colostomy would serve no purpose. In my opinion, we need to remove the whole of the large bowel, in other words, perform a panproctocolectomy. This operation means removing both rectum and colon. You would then have two options, a permanent ileostomy or an ileo-anal pouch.'

Hazel and I were speechless. We were just beginning to get used to the idea of a colostomy operation, but were now faced with either an ileostomy or an ileo-anal pouch. The surgeon was suggesting something radically different to a colostomy, something much larger and more serious.

The surgeon went on to explain that I would need to have another colonoscopy to provide an accurate and up-to-date reading of the condition of the colon and rectum. This would need to be done before he could suggest what the best option would be for me.

I was also to be referred to a stoma nurse; someone who specialised in colostomy and ileostomy operations. She would be able to talk us through the process and could also introduce us to people who had had similar operations to the one that I was about to undergo. They would be able to let us know their thoughts, both positive and negative, about what had happened to them.

A stoma care nurse is highly trained and is a senior nurse who is trained especially to work with stoma patients. Working alongside other nursing staff, they provide extra support during hospital stays and for when a patient returns home. For instance, he or she will introduce you to the first pouch you will wear in hospital.

We spent almost two hours with the stoma nurse, who patiently reassured us, helped us come to terms with the process of the operation and explained how we would manage afterwards. Hazel and I both found the time with the stoma nurse invaluable. We were reassured and encouraged. Every question that raced through our minds was answered. It was very comforting to know that we would receive her care before the operation. Advice would be given about various stoma appliances and where they might be sited on the abdomen. We were also to be told in detail how to prepare for the operation, the cleaning and care of the stoma, and other matters.

At this point I found out that an ileostomy is only performed when it is essential for the future well being of the patient. Inflammatory diseases of the colon, especially UC and Crohn's Disease, may be so profound that there is no alternative other than extremely radical surgery.

For some people the ileo-anal pouch operation is preferable to the permanent ileostomy, although it is not suitable for people who have Crohn's Disease. A downside of this operation is that inflammation of the pouch, known as pouchitis, can occur. Patients may feel unwell and have a high temperature and diarrhoea. There may also be occasional rectal bleeding. The problem can, however, be treated with antibiotics.

With this operation, there is a need for a temporary ileostomy in the first instance, which means having a temporary stoma. The surgeon forms a pouch in the patient. After two or three months the patient returns for surgery to have the ileo-anal pouch completed. This means there is no longer the need for a stoma. If the operation is not successful, however, a permanent ileostomy will be required.

We felt numb as the stoma nurse, patiently and gently, talked us through the whole process. We were told that arrangements would be made for us to meet two people in similar circumstances to myself. They would be people who had undergone surgery, one with a permanent ileostomy, the other with the ileo-anal pouch. We would be able to ask these people many questions that would be running through our minds. The answers would help to give us a more accurate assessment of the two operations, together with their advantages and disadvantages.

With assurances provided that the hospital would arrange for me to have a colonoscopy, we made the journey home. We tried very lamely to take in what we had just been told. Questions such as 'Why has this happened to me?' and 'How will we cope?' were very much to the fore.

Emotions fluctuated between panic and fear as we tried very hard to come to terms with the immediate future. We had left home expecting to discuss having a colostomy operation, but we were going home discussing the relative merits of a permanent ileostomy or an ileo-anal pouch. The concepts were at first too hard to grasp.

Before we left the hospital, we had been given brochures that provided in-depth information about both procedures, together with a sample stoma bag, to help us to come to terms with our future. Neither of us, however, could bring ourselves to look at the brochures, especially not the bag. We hadn't yet had enough time to come to terms with the fact that this was the way things would be from now on – unless God intervened with divine healing.

As the days went by, everything began to settle in our minds. If I were to say I wasn't fearful, I would be lying. The truth was I was terrified. It would be a complete change in my lifestyle, and one that would happen quite quickly.

By now we had read the literature about the operations and had looked, albeit briefly, at the bag we had been given. I found it very difficult to show this bag to anyone other than Hazel. It was a great psychological hurdle for me. Then one day my youngest daughter visited us. I had left the brochures on a table and had forgotten that I had secreted the bag inside one of them. She asked if she could look at the brochures and, before I realised it, the bag fell out into her lap. I was shocked. But she just laughed and started talking to me about it. From that day onwards I lost my embarrassment about this appliance.

People began praying for us, expecting a miracle, but there wasn't one. What did happen, though, is that we were filled with a very special peace. It was, I believe, the 'perfect peace' that 'surpasses all understanding' (Philippians 4:7). Isaiah 26:3 says 'You will keep him in perfect peace, whose mind is stayed on You because he trusts in You'. 'Perfect peace' is a term in Hebrew known as *shalom, shalom*. It emphasises our health and well being. It is my belief that if we trust in our Heavenly Father to help us on the way ahead He fills us with this Godly peace, enabling us to manage each situation as it arrives. It is when you know that, whatever happens, it will be all right. It is when the mind, rather than wandering off at a tangent, remains calm, with the knowledge that God is in control and is capable of sorting things out for us. This peace ensured that Hazel and I were able to face the future with a little more confidence. It did not happen all of a sudden. As far as I was concerned it came as I focused on the way ahead and faced the obstacles in my mind head on. I decided it was no use to deny what was going to happen. It *was* going to happen. I was not in a dream. This was reality and I needed to face up to the future because it was imminent.

The breakthrough in my acceptance of what was going to happen was in my facing the situation and involving God in it. As I focused on God and attempted to draw strength from Him, I had a wonderful feeling that everything would be all right. I could have left Him out. But the key to the peace I felt was calling out to Him and receiving His reassurance that everything would be all right.

God continued to speak to me. He gave me 1 Peter 4:12: 'Beloved, do not think it strange concerning the fiery trial which is to try you.' He reinforced the fact that I was not alone. He was with me and wanted me to be filled with courage. I knew that when He brought me out of the trial, I would know Him better, trust Him more and have something to say that could help people in similar situations to my own.

God helped me to see that even though the road ahead was difficult, I would manage to walk it. I would manage to cope with the difficult life in the future and be equipped with the confidence and reassurance to help others in need to see they could, too.

It was early days, however, and I knew I would need all of His strength and presence very soon in the future.

4

MIXED EMOTIONS

'It's the best thing that's happened to me – it's given me my life back!'

That appeared to be the thoughts of the two people I had spoken to about the surgery they'd had, one with an ileo-anal pouch and the other with a permanent ileostomy. Although they differed as to the relative merits regarding the two operations, the conclusion was the same: 'Once I didn't have a life – now I do.'

It was so wonderful to talk to people who knew exactly what I was going through. Even though Hazel understood a great deal about my suffering, she had no idea what it felt like because she herself hadn't experienced it. Neither had any of my friends or members of my family, except my eldest daughter and my mother. By this time my mother, who had very rarely talked about the disease, had died and my daughter lived a long way away from me so we never really had the chance to talk things through. To be face-to-face with other UC sufferers who were positive about the operations they had gone through was a real tonic. My surgeon insisted that his patients had these meetings as he maintained they helped them to face up to the operation and their future lifestyle.

Following such drastic surgery it would not be possible to resume a 'normal' life free from emotional upsets. But in any event, prior to any operation, a UC sufferer would not be living anything that could be described as normal, if 'normal' is defined as standard or usual. What can definitely be said, though, is that following this drastic surgery there is certainly a degree of improvement in the patient's quality of life, and over time the improvement may increase. Surgery, however, is a life-changing event, one that involves great psychological changes. Life can never be the same again.

Although I considered both operations carefully, I couldn't decide which would be best for me. I have never been very good at making decisions. In fact Hazel has often said she hoped her life never had to depend on my making a decision. I suppose that at the back of my mind I still hoped God would heal me – and then I wouldn't have to go through such an ordeal. I knew lots of people were praying for such healing but I already knew what I believed God had told me and that I really had only two options to consider.

There were mixed emotions. One part of me was gradually coming to accept an operation, although which operation was not yet clear. The other was willing God to turn up at the last moment like a hero from an action-packed movie. But no one could tell me what to do. If they had tried to do so they would have been setting themselves up for criticism should I have felt the need to blame someone later on. People could guide me and give their opinion, but at the end of the day any decision was down to me. I felt in such turmoil.

I didn't know what to expect. Although I'd read all the literature until I could practically recite it, I still didn't know what it would feel like after the operation. How would I feel? What would happen to me? Would I survive? So many things could go wrong.

I think the hardest thing to face up to was that, whatever I decided, I had to have an operation. Once I accepted that an operation was going to happen, I would then be able to concentrate on what operation to have and discuss the matter with the surgeon and stoma nurse. The decision, however, might not have to be taken by me following the colonoscopy. This might show that only one possible option was feasible.

I had a lot to think about, but as the days went on found I was able to face up to what was going to happen. I even began to re-read the brochures the hospital had given me, and eventually looked closely at the bag I'd been given.

Although it was a strange idea, the thought of having an ileostomy bag fitted to my stomach wall, albeit permanently or for a short time, didn't seem too dreadful. When I held the sample bag close to my body, it didn't appear too unsightly or cumbersome. I stood in front of the bedroom mirror trying to imagine what it would be like. Although it was too difficult to understand in detail, I did manage to get an idea. I decided it would not be unbearable. I actually wore the bag for a few days, trapped inside my pants, to get a better feel of what it was like. At first it felt peculiar, but after a while I forgot it was there. Psychologically this was a boost, because I was looking at it when I was undressed, and so was Hazel.

It made me think how difficult it must be for all those unfortunate people who have accidents (car crashes and the like) and who, because of the nature of their injuries, have to have emergency stoma surgery. These people don't have the benefit of any thinking time at all. One moment they are all right and the next transported to a lifestyle they have not in the least prepared for. It must be extremely distressing for the person who has the accident and for friends and family.

The letter finally arrived to let me know the date of the colonoscopy. Even though I was expecting it, it was still a jolt. I really did have to face up to everything now. I found out that I would need to go on a reduced diet for five days before the test. I would then need to take strong laxatives, followed by lots of water, to clear and flush out my system.

A colonoscopy is a test that allows a doctor to look at the lining of the colon. A colonoscope, a long, flexible tube, sufficient to travel the whole length of the colon and about the thickness of an index finger, is very carefully passed inch-by-inch through the anus into the colon, and then all the way round the bowel until it reaches the appendix. It has a bright light on one end with tiny forceps. The doctor has a clear view of the lining of the bowel when looking down the tube. An assessment can be made there and then as to whether or not there is any disease. A biopsy may also be taken by removing a piece of tissue with the forceps, which will then be sent for analysis. After the test, the surgeon will have a much clearer picture of the internal situation.

The day of the colonoscopy arrived and, having followed the low-residue diet very carefully and taken the laxatives, I was ready, albeit a little fearful, for the test.

Hazel drove me to the hospital and I very reluctantly walked into the endoscopy unit. I had had my last colonoscopy two years earlier and knew what to expect, but as a confirmed coward I was not looking forward to this particular procedure again.

After the preliminaries of signing consent forms, assuring the medical staff that I understood what the test was about and making sure I didn't want to go to the toilet, I was eventually shown into the room where the test was to be carried out.

It was rather like what you would expect an operating theatre to look like. There was medical equipment everywhere, and nurses and auxiliaries around me wiring up my hand for the sedation and taking my blood pressure. I felt it should have been rocketing by now, but as no one paid any particular interest in it, it must have been all right.

Once the surgeon came into the room I was given a sedative. Unlike the previous colonoscopy, when I had been out cold, this time what I was given only made me very sleepy. I was slightly aware of what was going on around me. What happened was a little uncomfortable, but with the help of the sedative I knew little about it.

Even though I was in theatre for over an hour, it seemed only minutes later that I was drinking a cup of tea (wonderful after so long) and trying to talk to Hazel.

I was able to talk to the surgeon, who confirmed that the colitis was severe and that surgery would be necessary. As I was still not sure what option to choose an appointment for six weeks ahead was made, and I left for home.

By now, the downstairs toilet that the social services had made sure I could have was well on the way to being completed, and there were builders and rubble everywhere. A downstairs toilet would very much help to give me a better quality of life. It would also be a great asset after my operation, as it would offer a place with the privacy and availability that I didn't have at the present time.

There is always a price to pay, however. In this case it was dust, dust and more dust. It was coming out of our ears; we could literally taste it. Everywhere we sat, walked or just perched had a coating of brick dust, and we lived like this for just over a week. In the long run, however, it was well worth the upheaval.

While the builders were building the toilet, I had plenty of time for reflection. I began to look at my situation in a little more depth. I was still waiting for a date for surgery and it seemed that it was God's will for me to endure this. He had offered no other solution in the guise of healing.

It was during this time that I felt God was reinforcing within me the message that, even though I had a disability, I had a purpose. God had a plan and a purpose for my life. Whether God took me out of the situation or took me through it, I had to trust Him because He was working for my good and for the good of those I might be able to help. I had an inner feeling that God was in control of things and that I was 'doing' His will. This greatly encouraged me as I waited for an appointment with the surgeon.

When we go through trials and tribulations, it is easy to focus only on one's self and forget our loved ones who stand by us in the midst of our suffering. Hazel was a great source of encouragement to me, and without her I'm sure I would never have survived. She had needs as well, however. She needed to talk to someone so that she could vent her feelings and share her burdens with a willing listener. Apart from family and friends there was no one. She had access to the stoma nurse and also knew my consultant's nurse, but she had no medical advisor whom she could talk to about her problems. My ill health was a great burden for her to carry, and one where she needed to lean heavily on God for her strength and sanity. There is a great need for more support groups, especially ones for UC sufferers' spouses and their nuclear families. Hazel had the greatest support in her Saviour and friend Jesus Christ, but she also needed to be with other carers of UC sufferers who understood exactly what she was going through.

I am sure that Hazel knew off by heart the verse 'Cast your cares on the Lord and He will sustain you; He will never let the righteous fall.' (Psalm 55:22), and used it as a daily resource. I do know that at this time God showered her with His grace and carried her through each day.

I heard nothing from the hospital. After a few weeks I decided to phone the stoma nurse to find out what was happening. She wanted to know if I'd made a decision about the type of surgery that I wanted. If I had, she was sure the surgeon would accept the decision, whatever I chose, which would mean I wouldn't have to see him again. I could then wait for a date for surgery.

The ileo-anal pouch seemed a good idea but I didn't relish the risk of pouchitis, that is, inflammation of the smaller bowel. Furthermore, I did not like the idea of having to empty my bowel five or six times a day, which I'd been told would have been necessary because of the lack of a colon. The lack of a colon would make the bowel movements quite loose and frequent. I also didn't want to have to have two, or possibly three, major operations if the first was not successful. I wanted everything over and done with, which is why I chose to have a bag and a permanent ileostomy. I would then be completely free of the disease. No more medication or hospital tests. No more pain and suffering. No more colitis.

I did, of course, have one other option, which was to have no operation. I did consider this, but came to the conclusion that, as I had not had a divine revelation from God Himself about the matter, it would be risky and somewhat foolish to do nothing as the end result might be disastrous.

I was told that the surgery would be in about six weeks' time, and that following the operation I would be in hospital for about two weeks. I would then be allowed home if it were thought I would be able to look after myself. I would, however, need to convalesce for about three months.

5

OFF TO HOSPITAL

Patience is not one of my virtues. Before long I was on tenterhooks waiting for a letter confirming the date of my operation.

The anxiety I suffered as each day went by without a letter arriving was very great but self-inflicted. Now that I had made my decision to go for a permanent ileostomy I wanted the operation over and done with. Anything that wasn't relevant to this I reckoned was holding me up and preventing me from having my life back.

After trying to cope with my fear and my procrastination for many months, the fact that major surgery was imminent was overwhelming. I was both apprehensive and impatient. The urgent need for the operation was not because I thought I might change my mind, however. That thought never occurred to me. Nevertheless I was fearful of the operation and wondered whether I would survive it.

In retrospect I think my impatience was totally selfish. I acted as if I was the only one who needed surgery. It was as if I was the only person in the world who, right at that moment, had to have the surgeon's undivided attention. I hang my head in shame at my thoughts at that time.

Even so, I reckon my reaction was probably typical. I felt I had suffered enough and now had the opportunity of having surgery that would give me a better quality of life. I wanted it immediately.

As a mature adult, however, I had to understand that I couldn't have things as and when I thought I needed them. I had to accept that there was a waiting period, hard though it was to accept this, and that there was a valid reason why the operation couldn't be carried out straight away. After all, I was not the only one waiting for stoma surgery.

As a Christian, I not only needed to realise this and be patient but also act in love in the process. I remembered that Psalm 37.7 says 'Rest in the Lord and wait patiently for Him.' I needed to be in a place of rest and peace where there is no place for impatience because my whole trust is in the Lord. He did not want me to be in a state of distress and anguish.

As I considered this verse of scripture, I became aware that it is so easy to act rudely by getting worked up and agitated. All this would accomplish would be to upset Hazel, my family and the medics who were trying to help me. It was so important for me to be in charge of what was happening to me, and it was essential to be so if I was to make my mark as a Christian in the world.

I was professing Christianity, in other words telling the world that I belonged to God. Acting in a brash, self-centred or impatient way, therefore, would not help to influence either people or circumstances positively. My behaviour would simply irritate or upset others. As I realised this, I began to accept the reality of the situation. The letter would come in good time, not when I demanded it. I would just have to wait, patiently.

I'm convinced God allowed the waiting period to teach me a lesson. I had to overcome my impatience. In hindsight I think I was being taught a valuable lesson, but at the time what I was learning was not easy and it was very stressful. I really had to grit my teeth to survive.

By now, the colitis was rampant and I could only manage to cope with short periods at a time. I had to plan each day carefully and decide in advance if I was going to be able to carry out particular tasks. Depression kicked in. Because UC was now taking over my life, it became very difficult to get through each day. The pain seemed to be getting much worse. Also, I had to keep on taking the medication, but it didn't seem to be doing any good. In fact it didn't seem to be doing anything except beat my body about with side effects. Even the retention enemas now failed to do their job properly. My rectum was so sore that it became almost impossible to insert them into my anus. If I did manage to do so, the liquid would come out again after a few minutes, making a great mess of everything.

I didn't know what to do or think. One moment I would try to rejoice and laugh myself through my messy, painful life. But the next I would be reduced to tears. Even though I'm a Christian and felt God's love and presence within me, it was an exceedingly difficult time to go through. I felt increasingly isolated as I became a virtual prisoner to my condition. At this time I leaned even more heavily on Jesus than I'd ever done before, seeking His comfort and help. I had nowhere and no one else I could turn to, except Hazel, and she had her own problems with caring for me. I firmly believed that God wanted me to be totally reliant upon Him. A Christian basically gives his or her life to Jesus. It is not that Christians have their own free will taken away from them; they choose to give up their free will and instead carry out God's will.

For me as a Christian and in my miserable condition, I felt that God wanted me to turn to Him for help because I had decided to be His child when I became a Christian. I believed He had the answers to my many questions and my best interests at heart. It was a matter of faith and trust in God. I was not angry with Him for leaving me in such pain and misery and knew that ultimately He would help me through my suffering. And sometimes, even in great pain, I was able to be at peace.

'The postman's here,' Hazel called out to me.

My heart sank as I picked up the letter. I had waited so long for this moment. It had been just over three months since I'd decided on the permanent ileostomy, although it had seemed more like six. Now I'd got what I wanted, immediately I didn't want it.

I knew the letter was from the hospital and yet froze at the thought of opening it. The letter stated the time and date (13 November 2000) to attend the hospital for the long-awaited surgery. It was surgery that would give me a new lease of life. Yet here I was in a state of blind panic.

I had to go to the hospital several days before my operation for the pre-clerking procedure. This involved completing consent forms, giving details of my past medical history, having my blood pressure taken and talking through the implications and practicalities of hospital procedure.

I was filled with unexpected emotions. One moment I was elated at the prospect of being relieved of my condition so that I could get on with my life. The next I was angry, frightened and bewildered. I think these mixed emotions are probably common to all those who are about to undergo major surgery. It's perhaps part of having to deal with a big change in our lives.

The day finally arrived. Following a telephone call to check that the bed was still available, we made our way to the hospital. I wanted the journey to last forever, but there was no traffic to hold us up so that within a very short time Hazel had pulled up the car at the main door of the hospital.

We booked in at the main desk on the surgical ward and were told that there would be a slight delay as there had been an emergency. This gave me time to marshal my thoughts and familiarise myself with the hospital surroundings and escape routes. The ward I was to be in appeared very busy with people walking about everywhere. I tried to read but couldn't concentrate. I tried to talk to Hazel but didn't know what to say. We had said everything we felt we needed to say to each other before we arrived. I filled in the time by walking up and down the corridor for what seemed to be a very long time until the nursing staff were ready for me and I was shown to my bed.

I had had to wait for perhaps an hour, and although this had somewhat helped me to familiarise myself with my new surroundings, it was nevertheless a long wait and one that was very stressful.

Hazel left, and I unpacked the few things I had with me and waited. I didn't have long to wait. The staff nurse returned with some strong-acting laxative called Picolax. This mixture contains sodium picosulphate, a stimulant. It works by increasing the activity of the intestine. It also contains magnesium citrate, an osmotic laxative that helps the bowel to retain a certain amount of fluid so that later it can be flushed out effectively.

The Picolax is dissolved in water and at once becomes extremely hot. Water is added to the solution before it is drunk. The drink seemed to have an orange flavour and wasn't all that bad. The Picolax is administered twice. The effects are slow at first but later extremely effective, the result being endless trips to the loo. But this, of course, was routine for me. I was also given a bottle of orange drink to dilute in water, as a lot of liquid had to be consumed over the next twelve hours or so, together with a nutritionally complete blackcurrant drink, which in my opinion was disgusting. This was to make sure there were a constant level of nutrients in my body. I myself would sooner have had a cup of tea, but after a certain time tea was not allowed.

I was in a ward with five other people who occasionally glanced over in my direction and nodded at me. I'm a private person and would have preferred a room of my own, but at least I was in a corner. At this stage I was still dressed in my day clothes and seemed a little out of place. I had to remain dressed until after the stoma nurse had been to see me, as she needed to see me fully clothed. By seeing where the belt-line, underpants and trousers hang on a patient's body, the stoma nurse can accurately assess the correct site for the stoma and bag. This is an exacting procedure and needs to be done with considerable care to avoid leakage at a later stage. There have to be no folds or creases in the skin where the stoma is to be sited. It was also necessary to think about the type of trousers and underpants I would be wearing in the future. I also had to consider where the waistband might fall and whether it would impede the smooth functioning of the bag.

The stoma nurse drew with an ordinary permanent black marker pen on the wall of my stomach where the surgeon was to site the stoma and a sticky protector was placed over the area drawn on to stop it being wiped off. I briefly discussed the operation with her, and what my life would be like immediately after the operation and for the forthcoming months. After our talk I felt more reassured and decided to try to settle into where I was going to be for the following two weeks.

My temperature and blood pressure were taken at regular intervals, but other than that I was left to my own devices for the rest of the day. I got out of my day clothes and into my pyjamas, something I was pleased about as I was beginning to feel rather conspicuous in a ward full of other patients. I was glad to join in the dress code.

I had to wear surgical stockings. These fit very tightly, and need to be put on by someone who knows how to do this. The stockings only come up to the knees and are so tight they threaten to stop the blood flowing through the veins. They are essential to wear before a major operation, however, as they help prevent thrombosis. But fashion-wise they do nothing for the wearer and I think make one's feet feel sweaty and very cold. It's funny lying around while someone struggles to put them on.

In the evening I had to prepare for the operation the following day by shaving my stomach and groin. The shaving was required to help the surgeon to do his job properly. I also had to shave my left thigh in case I needed to be 'shocked' (that is, resuscitated) whilst in surgery and under the anaesthetic. This was an extremely sobering thought.

With preparations for the operation completed, apart from a final shower before the operation the following morning, I tried to settle down. I thought I would relax with a crossword book I had brought with me. I attempted to alter the level of the pillows by adjusting the backrest, but the backrest crashed and disappeared down the back of the bed, smashing against the floor. Everyone looked at me with a start. Even patients from the ward next door that looked on to mine were staring at me, as were the nurses from the nurse's station outside. At that moment I wanted the ground to swallow me up I was so embarrassed.

I kept a low profile for the rest of the evening. In between dashing out to the loo, because the laxative was now beginning to work very effectively, I busied myself with crosswords. Just before lights out, a nurse reminded me that I had to shower before surgery in the morning and I tried to settle myself down for the night, my mind racing with the thought that I would be the first to go down for surgery the following day.

I couldn't sleep. My mind wouldn't shut down. One moment I was thinking about the positive aspects of the operation; the next minute focusing on the negative aspects wondering if everything would be all right. I must have checked a dozen times to see if the mark where the stoma was to be was still on my stomach. I would rub my hand over the site, wondering what it would feel like with the stoma in place. I couldn't imagine it. Fear tried to take a grip but at the same time I knew full well that it was now much too late to change my mind and stop having the surgery that I had waited so long for. It was now time to face up to it. All these many thoughts were rushing through my head as I gradually drifted into a very light sleep.

6

FROM DESPAIR TO MIRACLE

'Come on Mr Howard,' sounded the voice of the staff nurse, breaking into the only hour's sleep that I had had all night. 'It's time to have your shower and get ready for surgery.'

I lay in my hospital bed wondering where on earth I was and what I was doing. Then everything came back to me in a flash. It was Tuesday 14 November 2000. I was in hospital and was going to have major surgery in just over an hour's time.

I shot out of bed and made my way to the bathroom. The Picolax was still working and the results needed to be dealt with quickly. I also needed to shower and get back to bed for the pre-med I'd asked for, to calm me down before the operation.

Hospitals are usually warm, very warm, but this particular morning the shower room was freezing. Someone had left the window wide open. With a hard frost outside, the warm room had been transformed into a walk-in refrigerator. I quickly shut the window and let the steaming hot water warm and somewhat invigorate my freezing cold body.

I could have stayed in the shower all day long, but time was pressing and I needed to return to the ward as soon as possible.

The pre-med was given to me as a tablet. After that my memory of events is rather vague. I remember a porter pushing my bed along the corridor and I think a nurse accompanied us. I know we entered a lift and that the journey finished in what I presume was the operating theatre. There appeared to be lots of people around me working at top speed. All the time someone was talking to me, explaining what was going to happen. The explanation was in vain, however, as I didn't care about anything and in any event wouldn't have understood what being said. Then everything went dark and I became unconscious once the anaesthetic had taken effect.

The first thing I remember when I gradually became conscious after the operation was being in a strange place. I had started out in a large ward but was now in a little room with a nurse, who was attending to something or other. There was someone sitting at my side and at first I found it difficult to focus on who this might be. After a little while I realised it was Hazel; I recognised her beige fleece jacket. I was so pleased to see her I began to cry. She was her usual wonderful self and gently comforted me, telling me that everything had gone well.

For the first few hours after the operation I drifted in and out of sleep. This couldn't have been much fun for Hazel. During the late afternoon I was a little more coherent and Hazel began to tell me about what had happened. Apparently I'd been in the operating theatre for over four hours and had then spent a considerable time in the recovery room. I don't remember anything about this, only that I felt extremely cold. Hazel told me the bag the surgeon had placed on the stoma had come off and that I had had to be cleaned up. I had, however, been oblivious to all this.

I gradually began to get my bearings and realised I was in a small room next to the main ward. It looked out on to a pleasant grassed area, had a television and remote control and its own washing facilities. This was all I needed, really. Not that I could enjoy any of these facilities at the time. I was wired up to a drip that was housed on a tall trolley with electronic meters on it. I had a drain in my stomach and a catheter fitted to my penis to drain the urine, as well as an epidural in my back to help me cope with the pain. Other tubes and drains were fitted in my hands and arms and an oxygen mask was fitted over my nose and mouth. I had metal clips in my stomach, rather like staples. These were used to seal up the nine-inch incision that the surgeon had made in my stomach in order to carry out the operation. I felt like a Frankenstein creation.

My anus had been stitched up. My rectum and sphincter muscles had been removed along with the whole of my colon, so the anus was therefore now surplus to requirements. As there was no longer any gut connected to my anus it needed to be closed up to prevent infection. A stoma had been created with my ileum. My ileum had been brought out on to the stomach wall and the end bit had been formed into a stoma. From now on I would be using the stoma to get rid of all bodily waste, as there was no longer a colon to carry the waste through to the rectum.

For some days after my operation, I fluctuated between high and low temperatures. I had hot and cold sweats and felt quite dreadful. One moment I would feel all right, the next cold and shaky. I had a raging thirst. The sign above my bed said 'Nil by mouth'. I could see people walking by with cups of tea and cold drinks. Some auxiliaries came into my room and asked if I'd like a cup of tea. This was agony, as I had to say no. They were obviously not familiar with my condition.

The stoma nurse visited me. Hazel was there when she checked my stoma. When she saw it, Hazel looked at me, clearly shocked, and said, 'What have they done to you?' We were both overwhelmed and shed a few tears. The tears to some extent released our extremely pent up emotions, thus drawing us closer together and also giving me much more confidence about letting Hazel see the stoma. As she was going to look after me this was essential.

A physiotherapist visited me not long afterwards. Her job was to help me breathe properly to clear my lungs and to show me how to protect my stomach by placing my hands on it if I coughed or sneezed suddenly. She told me she would be back in a few days time to help me walk about. The way I felt then made me think I would never be able to do this. My weakness was overwhelming.

On the day following the operation, I was visited by one of the surgeon's assistants. She asked if anyone had told me what had been found during the operation.

'What do you mean? What had been found?' I asked panic-stricken. 'What was found?'

'Colitis,' she replied. 'The colon was completely riddled with UC, right up to your appendix, which was ready to erupt. We had to remove your appendix as well. It was thought we should send the colon away for further analysis.'

'Was there anything nasty in there?' I asked fearfully.

'We can't rule out cancer at this stage,' replied the assistant, 'but try not to worry. We'll have the results back within five working days.'

'Try not to worry,' I thought as she made her way out of the room. 'What does she expect me to do?'

I was in a strange environment and felt absolutely dreadful. I had no one to comfort or support me, as Hazel was at home. I had just been told something that was frightening and uncertain. I felt scared and began to fret about what the doctor had said. Yes I was a Christian and yes I did believe I would have eternal life, meaning that if I died I believed I would go to Heaven. But I was not ready to go, not just yet. I became very tearful and started to panic. I was in a room by myself. I felt very alone.

Just then, my consultant's nurse came to see how I was. I felt so relieved when I first saw her I couldn't talk for crying.

When the nurse eventually understood what I'd just been told, she immediately reassured me.

'Don't be alarmed,' she said. 'There was no cancer to be seen when you had the colonoscopy. Although the investigation didn't pick up the UC in the appendix, I'm certain there's no tumour to worry about. Try not to think about it too much. I'll see if I can get an early result from the lab and I'll let you know what it is as soon as I find out.' With that she left me with the promise she'd be back soon. I was left to my own thoughts. I decided I was going to try not to think too negatively. I felt too weak and ill.

By Thursday, the second day after the operation, the doctors told me I could go on 'Sips'. This meant I was allowed to take extremely small sips of water every hour. This was sheer bliss, but now the desire to take a long and fulfilling drink was even greater than before. Unfortunately it seemed that it was too soon for liquid to be allowed into my system. I began to be violently sick and was relegated once again to 'Nil by mouth'. Over the next five days I alternated between 'Sips' and 'Nil by mouth' and began to despair. As soon as I felt I was beginning to make a little headway I was knocked back and became sick. What I vomited was actually more bile than anything else as there was very little of anything in my stomach. It was revolting. I think the thought of it will haunt me for the rest of my life.

No one can say they enjoy being sick. It is one of the most horrible things that we occasionally have to go through. Over the first five days or so after the operation, I probably vomited more than I had ever done before in the whole of my life. It was uncontrollable. I was given something to stop the vomiting but it made very little difference. I somehow had to get through what I was going through. I had a very bad time.

It was now Monday 20 November, six days after the operation. I was still nauseous and appeared to be making very little progress. I felt despair and frustration. People were praying for me and my pastor, Paul White, was visiting almost daily, but I didn't seem to be healing. I began to feel very depressed and I think that at that moment if I'd been able to press a self-destruct button I would have done so. I felt so weak, thirsty and helpless. Part of me wondered if I would ever begin to feel well again. I would have been able to cope better if I'd been able to stop the nausea. Nevertheless, even during this period there were moments when I felt reasonably calm.

Hazel came to see me that morning. The stoma nurse was going to talk us through what was happening, and help me drain and change my bag. This was something I would have to get used to doing from now on for the rest of my life. Up until now the nursing staff had been dealing with the bag.

The stoma nurse gave me a bag of supplies that included spare bags, wipes, scented disposable bags and a blow-up cushion for me to sit on. This would help to alleviate the discomfort I was feeling from the stitched-up wound in my anus.

I managed so well with changing my bag that the stoma nurse was quite surprised. Quite early on, however, I had realised and accepted the fact that the bag was for life. I could either hate it or be positive about the necessary appliance and turn it into a 'not so bad' situation. I had chosen to be positive and by doing this found I learnt how to use the bag quite quickly.

The stoma nurse left and Hazel got a bottle of olive oil out of her handbag. She told me that the Colonel, a friend and colleague from our church, had said that he had felt that God had given him some scriptures and he thought they were relevant for me. He had told Hazel she should anoint me with oil, along with everything else in my little room. She should then pray some scriptures over me. The scriptures were to do with healing and anointing with oil. The olive oil has no particular qualities or power, other than that it is supposed to be pure. Hazel envisaged that the anointing of oil would offer God's protection to whatever it was applied to. In the Christian religion it is believed that people receiving healing should be anointed with oil by rubbing or smearing it on the person to be healed. Also, that external surfaces near the person requiring healing, if anointed with the same oil, provide protection for the person anointed.

I felt so weak that I paid little attention to what Hazel was doing. She anointed almost everything in sight. I'm sure that if anyone had walked in at that moment, she would have put some oil on him or her as well. She wiped it on the doorposts, the handles, the window frames, the bed … and me. It was everywhere: wall-to-wall anointing. All the time as she did this she was praying out loud.

With all that anointing it might have been thought that I would have been healed instantly, but I wasn't. Actually, I began to feel worse.

Hazel left not long afterwards and I tried to get some rest. Soon afterwards, however, I was violently sick again. The nurses had to change my clothes and some of the bedding. I lay in my bed, burning hot. On my bedside table was a jug of iced water. I reached out, dipped my fingers in to it and wiped them over my forehead to cool me down. At that moment I felt the need to make the sign of the cross on my forehead with the cold water. I did not know why, it just felt the right thing to do. I called out to God to help me. I reminded Him that I was His child and that I had been anointed with oil.

I drifted off into sleep for a while, and it was almost as if I felt God saying

'Get your hands off him Satan. He's mine!'

The physiotherapist woke me up. She had come to see if I would like to go for a walk around the ward. I said I would and she agreed to give me a few minutes to wake up. Somehow I felt better. Something had happened during that short sleep. I cannot really say how, but I had a fresh determination to be more positive about my situation. I got out of bed and although I felt dreadfully weak and wobbly, I was standing up ready for the physiotherapist on her return. She took me down the corridor and was surprised at how I managed to walk. I walked the length of the corridor before going back to my room and on my return I didn't get back in bed but sat in a chair.

I was in the chair when Hazel returned. I sat there reading a book and although I felt weak I was also determined that things were going to be better from now on. I was put back on to 'Sips' and this time resolved to take everything very slowly.

Quite suddenly I began to make a rapid recovery. At first Hazel couldn't believe what was happening. I started to watch television, something I hadn't had the slightest interest in doing during the previous week. I also walked with Hazel down to the main reception when she left the hospital.

As I sat up in bed that evening a verse of scripture came into my head. When I looked it up it read, 'My horn (strength), You have exalted like a wild ox; I have been anointed with fresh oil' (Psalm 92:10). I was truly astonished. It was as if God was telling me to remember this whenever things started to go wrong. If ever I began to feel ill I could quote this verse and claim that I had been strengthened and anointed with fresh oil, thus reminding and encouraging myself that I had been healed. I was amazed and very blessed by this thought. It helped me a great deal during the rest of my stay in hospital and indeed it still does today.

A week after my operation, I was walking all over the hospital. By now the drips, painkillers, drains and catheter had gone and I was free to move around. I was not on any medication. Apart from feeling sore and still with a fluctuating temperature I felt all right. I was, of course, still very weak and very light-headed, but I had a new-found determination that had not been there before. From thereon, I believe God helped me to heal and that it was His love, grace and compassion that gave me the willpower to get on with my life.

I had received many get-well cards. They all meant so much to me, but there was one that particularly affected me. Jenny, who was in my Home group (a small group of church people who meet at our home), sent one with the message 'Read Psalm 121. It's for you, Grahame.'

The Psalm reads as follows:

> *'I will lift up my eyes to the hills,*
> *From whence comes my help?*
> *My help comes from the Lord*
> *Who made Heaven and earth.*
>
> *He will not allow your foot to be moved*
> *He who keeps you will not slumber*
> *Behold He who keeps Israel*
> *Shall neither slumber nor sleep.*
>
> *The Lord is your keeper*
> *The Lord is your shade*
> *At your right hand*
> *The sun shall not strike you by day*
> *Nor the moon by night*
>
> *The Lord shall preserve you*
> *From all evil*
> *He shall preserve your soul.*
> *The Lord shall preserve your*
> *Going out and your coming in*
> *From this time forth and even*
> *Forevermore.'*

The Psalm deeply affected me. It was a reminder that only God could rescue me. I believed then and believe now that as I call out to Him He is there and will send the help that I need.

The following day I was moved to the main ward. I had mixed emotions about this. Although this was progress, in the room by myself I had been alone with my thoughts. Now other people would surround me. Regardless of what I thought, however, the move had to take place. I was now drinking coffee and tea but was not yet eating any food.

7

BACK HOME

'I think you can start on a little food, Mr Howard,' said a doctor once he had finished examining me. 'Take it easy at first, but I think you'll be fine now.'

I nodded my thanks and appreciation as he left. I hadn't eaten anything for ten days and was famished.

The day before, having moved back into the main ward, I felt I was undergoing torture watching other patients eat. Now at last I could eat and I wanted to enjoy my food, and enjoy it immediately. Fortunately I didn't have to wait long. Even though breakfast had finished a long time previously, a nurse, bless her, brought me some cornflakes, toast and marmalade, along with a cup of coffee. It was sheer bliss. I took my time. I didn't want to be sick again and have to revert back to not eating. It must have taken me about an hour to eat the meal, but eat it I did and loved it.

At this stage no one had explained to me in detail what I could and couldn't eat.

I had read various brochures that all seemed to suggest that I could eat what I liked. If some food didn't agree with me I should cut it down, but I was not to stop having it altogether. I had to eat slowly, keeping my mouth shut as I chewed, and was advised not to speak whilst eating. This was so I could digest the food properly and also to ensure that very little wind got into my system. It was not easy for me to do this as I had always liked to eat fast, and sometimes I gulped food down. I also found it difficult at times to stop talking when I ate, which was not good for my limited digestive system. This would be another minor problem I would have to contend with.

I had to really take in the fact that I didn't have a colon any longer and that my body would have to learn to cope only with the use of the smaller bowel and stoma. The surgery had led to the removal of my colon, rectum and sphincter muscles. I had been left with my small bowel and my ileum had been brought out on to my abdomen to form the stoma. This meant that I would need to try to eat easily digestible foods. I was anxious to avoid a blockage in my newly arranged gut, as this would mean an emergency trip to the hospital for a possible further operation. It would take a little time and practice to get used to the new arrangement. Nevertheless I reckoned that eventually it would be worth it in the end, as many had previously testified.

I began to think about going home. Actually I began to dream about going home and would constantly walk down the corridor towards the main entrance as if I were plotting my escape. Outside the weather was cold, wet and windy, and all around looked pretty dismal, but I longed to be out there. I hadn't had any fresh air since I'd been in hospital, apart from an open window, and I kept on imagining what it would be like to feel it on my face.

I decided not to go down the stairs and into the reception area. I would save that wonderful moment for my discharge that I hoped would be very soon. All around me people were dashing up and down the stairs and disappearing down the corridors. Life seemed to be lived at a fast pace in a hospital. I found this quite strange. Before my operation I'd been used to this type of lifestyle. Right now, though, I felt like someone aged ninety.

My consultant's nurse came to see me. She told me the test results had come through and that there was no sign of any malignancy. I could have kissed her. What I actually did was to cry. I cried with relief and gratitude to God for having answered my prayers. I had waited patiently for these results. I had refused to go down the road of gloom and doom, but this had not been easy. The relief was now amazing and I wanted to shout, very loudly.

I stood at the top of the stairs waiting to surprise Hazel. I didn't have long to wait. She almost walked by, as she hadn't expected to see me there. It was a sure sign that I was getting stronger and I hoped I would be discharged at the weekend. Some of the nurses, including one of the stoma nurses, had said this might be possible. I blurted out the good news about the test results to Hazel and was crying before I'd finished telling her. So was she. It was a very special moment as we hugged each other.

My temperature continued to fluctuate. One minute it would be all right; the next either high or below normal. This was frustrating because otherwise I was making excellent progress.

A day later when one of the doctor's was doing his rounds, he said: 'I think we'll take the clips out of your stomach today, Mr Howard, but the stitches in your bottom will have to wait until next week.'

'Will I have to come back to the hospital to have them out?' I asked. 'Or will the district nurse visit me?'

'What do you mean?' he replied. 'You're going nowhere until at least the middle of next week.'

With that, he walked out of the ward. I was devastated. All my hopes and dreams of going home that weekend had just been wiped out. I started to slip into despair, but quickly became angry. I managed to suppress the anger, however, and stomped off to the bathroom to drain my appliance and have a good moan to God about this latest set back.

'Now listen, Lord,' I complained, 'the doctors are messing me about. The nurses have said I could possibly go home this weekend, and yet the doctor I've just seen has said that I can't. Please sort this mess out, Lord. I don't think it's fair.'

This was a child speaking to his father. This is what I was doing. But I was speaking to my Heavenly Father; I was doing what His Word tells us to do: 'Cast your burden upon the Lord, And he shall sustain you' (Psalm 55:22). I had decided long ago that God was my Father, and that His word was true and that it contains many promises that we can believe in. I believe that when we are in trouble or need help we can call on Him. He will answer, but the answer may not be what we expect it to be. That is part of what it means to be committed to Him, to do His will, whatever the cost. This should not stop us from calling out to Him. That was what I was doing and I trusted Him enough to know that He would sort out my troubles for me, because I knew He had my best interests at heart.

I went back to the ward and within thirty minutes the surgeon came round with the same doctor I'd seen before, together with various other medical staff. I'd seen the surgeon most days since I'd been in hospital but we'd only had the briefest of talks about how I was coping after the operation. Now he said he wanted to examine me to check the metal clips in my stomach and the stitches where my anus had been.

He confirmed the former decision to remove the clips forthwith. He then asked me to roll over on to my side and checked the stitches in my anus. What he said next astonished me.

'The stitches in the backside can come out today as well.' Then, turning to the nurse, 'Now, how's he getting on with the bag? Is he managing it by himself?'

The nurse confirmed I was and so did I, which reinforced what the stoma nurse had been telling me about my ability to care for myself.

'That's good,' continued the surgeon. 'All right, home tomorrow.' And with that he walked out of the ward.

Once again, I was amazed. This time at the speed at which it seemed that God had answered my prayers. One minute I'd been told I couldn't go home until the following week, then, following a moan to my Father, I was going home tomorrow morning. My head spun with God's goodness.

A nurse came to me shortly afterwards, carrying a pair of pliers. Everyone in the ward looked at me as she pulled the curtain around the bed.

'Just going into the torture chamber,' I joked with one of the onlookers.

It was not too difficult to remove the clips. The wound had healed and in the process of healing had partially lifted the clips out. All the nurse had to do was give them a little tweak with the pliers. Although the thought sounds rather horrible it was in fact a fairly painless operation.

The stitches, however, were different. I think that stitches always hurt when they are extracted. Today was no exception, but the thought of going home the next day helped me bear the discomfort.

With the removal of the clips and stitches the rest of the day was my own. I told everyone I saw that I was going home. I was like a child expecting a new toy and couldn't keep the joy to myself. The world needed to know. If I could have had the fact featured on the national news I would have agreed to this, such was my elation. After eleven days there was now light at the end of a very long, dark tunnel and I felt good.

That day I had many visitors, all of whom had to hear my news. By the evening I had worn myself out with enthusiasm and had to lie on the bed for a rest. The temperature outside had dropped and I began to get cold. Hazel put some extra blankets on me and I drifted off into a pleasant doze.

'Mr Howard,' said a nurse waking me from my oblivion, 'I've got to take your temperature and blood pressure.'

I sleepily opened my mouth for the thermometer paper.

'You've got a temperature!' she exclaimed. 'It's quite high. You won't be going home tomorrow unless that goes down.'

'It must be all the blankets on me,' I replied defensively. 'I got quite cold and my wife piled them on me.'

'I shouldn't think so,' said the nurse as she walked out of the ward having recorded the temperature on my chart.

I watched her as she made her way up to the staff nurse. I could have sworn she was enjoying the situation. Again I talked to God, telling Him how I might be the victim of a false thermometer reading. I asked Him to let me have my temperature taken again.

The staff nurse came in a few minutes later and expressed concern at my high temperature. I told her I had been cold and that my wife had piled extra blankets on the bed. I asked her if she would consider taking my temperature again in five minutes time. To my astonishment she agreed. When she did so it was normal. I decided to stay away from extra blankets, at least until I had returned home.

I believe that without God's help I would have had to accept the first thermometer reading. I thanked God about a dozen times for helping me and was still thanking Him as I drifted off into sleep.

I awoke bright and early the next morning, Saturday 25 November. Discharge day I thought to myself as I drank a cup of tea. I rushed off to the bathroom, emptied my appliance and got myself ready to go. Hazel was coming for me at 10 a.m. 'Three hours to go,' I said to myself as I walked back into the ward. I busied myself getting my things out of the bedside locker. That took all of five minutes and I then had to sit and wait. I had no clothes with me and so couldn't get dressed. All I could do was wait. And I waited and waited until I was fed up with waiting.

At last, Hazel arrived and after what seemed forever I was allowed to go. Hazel told me later that I practically ran down the corridor to the main entrance. I just wanted to get away and get back to where I felt I belonged.

I managed the journey home rather well, although I was a little sore. I sat on the cushion that the stoma nurse had loaned me while Haze drove. It was refreshing being driven in the car and it made a welcome change from the frenetic world of the hospital. I insisted she drove the 'scenic' route home. This was a lovely quiet road that went through the heart of the Dorset countryside. The main road was too much hustle and bustle. Even before the operation I hadn't been able to manage it very well and I knew that now I wouldn't be able to cope with all the stopping and starting.

Eventually we arrived home. Our dog Chips was so pleased to see me. Hazel had to make sure that he didn't jump up, however, as that could have been quite painful, especially if he'd caught me in my stomach. The poor dog had been depressed since I'd been in hospital. Hazel had taken him to the vet as he had been moping about the place with no interest in anything. The vet had said he would improve when I came home, and he was right. Chips was as elated as I was.

I was so thrilled to get back home. All the people from the hospice that I now work in who go home say the same: 'I can't wait until I get home.' I know from experience how they feel.

Hazel had everything in place. I was to sit in an armchair with the special cushion the stoma nurse had given me. When I became tired I could go to bed to rest for a while and the district nurse was to visit every day to make sure the wounds in my abdomen and anus were healing properly.

I soon began to think about what I should or could be doing. That was a problem. My body had been beaten about a lot. My mind, however, was as active as ever and I really wanted to get on with things. But Hazel soon put a stop to that. I anyway don't think I could have done much. I was so weak and drained of physical energy. It took a tremendous effort just to sit in the chair and talk or watch television.

As I had lost a lot of weight I was often cold. The heating was on high but I just couldn't get warm and sat for most of the first day home covered with blankets. I soon settled in, however. I hadn't realised in the lead-up to the operation just how much it would take out of me. I felt like an old man. When I looked in the mirror this confirmed what I felt. But I was home and things could only get better from now on. Even though I felt as though I'd had a quarrel with a Chieftain tank, I was feeling positive and very pleased to be back.

Hazel, however, was not so sure. Unlike me she didn't like to rush things. As much as she wanted me back home she would have preferred that the doctors had agreed before I was discharged. She knew that I had pushed to be discharged. She was worried about things going wrong. Whilst in hospital I had been cared for by the clinical staff. At home, Hazel, although she had support from the stoma and district nurses, would be very much on her own.

She may well have been worried that she wouldn't be able to cope. After all, the situation was just as new to Hazel as it was to me. She was going to have to learn very fast and with hardly any support from other people. For many months she had thought and planned how she would manage to look after me. Now she was actually experiencing the managing. She began to be a little fearful and felt more than a little uncertain about how things would develop.

8

WORKING THROUGH THE HANGUPS

I found the move from hospital to home fairly manageable. I had more privacy and could be myself, in that I didn't feel I had to talk to anyone if I didn't want to and didn't have to be on my best behaviour. But realising that I was now on my own with no nurses or a doctor to support me was worrying at first. Having been in hospital for nearly a fortnight I might well have thought I couldn't cope without them. I reminded myself, however, that I did have a district nurse coming in every day to check my wounds and general health. My stoma care nurse visited me each week and I could phone her if I needed to. I also had Hazel who was with me all the time who looked after me, cooked my meals and kept me going.

I worried about Hazel as the situation was a tremendous strain on her. She had been with me through everything: the colitis and the resultant trauma, then the operation and the worry of how it would all turn out. A short while after I came home she managed to get out a little. This was mostly down to the church to see her friends or do the shopping. Getting out of the house perhaps gave Hazel a temporary respite but otherwise she had no support.

Coming home was hard for me at first in some ways. I quickly became tired and spent most afternoons dozing upstairs. Also I found I needed to go to bed at about 6.30 p.m.

Each day, however, I grew stronger and concentrated on

adjusting to my new life. It was wonderful not to have to keep dashing to the lavatory every few minutes. When I had UC a great deal of my time had been taken up with using the toilet. Initially it was quite strange to realise that this would no longer be the case, because I no longer had the disease. Previously I not only had pain but the anxiety of wondering if I would get to a toilet in time. Now at least I was free from both these worries. Even so there were a number of issues related to the operation that I had to work through. Although I'd thought a great deal about these issues before the operation, now that I'd had it I had to face up to their reality.

First I had to get used to the idea that I carried a label: 'Physically Disabled'. Being registered as physically disabled meant I had to think long and hard about being stigmatised. But who was stigmatising me? There was in fact no one I could point to and say 'That person is stigmatising me.' I was the same person I was before the operation, in fact rather more mobile and certainly healthier than before. The stigma was not a fact; it was a mental attitude of mine and I had to eradicate it by using my mind.

That I was physically disabled was a fact. The operation I'd had, that is, a permanent ileostomy with the complete removal of colon and rectum, is a recognised disability in Dorset. I have a blue card stating that I am registered as physically disabled. (Local councils do not always, however, agree on what constitutes physical disability, particularly as regards UC and the same or similar operation to the one I had. So it is important to contact your local authority to find out whether or not you are regarded as physically disabled. Following an operation for a permanent ileostomy you might possibly not know about being registered as physically disabled. In my case, as I had received help from the DSS to build a disabled toilet in my home, I was known to them so it was easy to be registered.)

Being registered as physically disabled did not confer any

particular advantages for me after my operation, except to reinforce the need for renewal of my blue disabled parking badge. It didn't, for example, qualify me for disability living allowance from the DSS.

Although physically disabled, I wasn't worried as far as employment was concerned, as I was self-employed. If, however, you are in full-time employment, It would make sense to let your employer know about your condition and your possible needs, and to explain that at times it may be necessary to go to the lavatory to change or drain the stoma bag. This is especially important if there has been an accident or if the appliance leaks or comes off. Although this doesn't usually happen you should always be alert to the possibility that it might.

Your place of work should have disabled facilities installed so it would be a good idea to say you will be using them, and why. Someone with an ileostomy or colostomy doesn't have a visible disability like others who are wheelchair-bound, nevertheless having a stoma is just as much a disability and you deserve the right to use the facilities provided. If you explain your situation this will go a long way to help to alleviate future problems. I have often received an odd look from someone if I've used a disabled toilet. At first I used to feel very guilty about this; I thought I should limp or do something else to suggest I was physically disabled as I walked away. After thinking about this, however, I decided that as I had been through a major, life-changing operation I had earned the right to use disabled facilities, and that I didn't have to pretend I had any further disablement no matter what looks I got.

If you are unemployed because you are ill, the DSS need to know this. Initially I was on sick leave from my job as a social worker for six months. During this time I received sick pay from the DSS. I then had to take ill-health retirement and received both a lump sum and a monthly pension. I claimed incapacity benefit for sixteen months until I started to work on a self-employed, part-time basis of two to three days weekly until my operation in November 2000. I found the DSS were very helpful. They did not pressurise me in any way. I think that because I was honest and up front with them they recognised that I was a genuine case and offered as much help as I needed. Some people very much dislike the DSS and I have heard people say they use Gestapo tactics to assess need. This is a strong and possibly unfounded assertion. If required the DSS can offer advice about retraining, or can try to help find a vacancy that is tailor-made for a particular disability.

There were money worries that I had to think through. I also had to be careful not to spend too much all at once. I took ill-health retirement in December 1988 and in addition to the pension I was given three months' tax-free salary that helped very much. With the addition of incapacity benefit for the sixteen-month period before I started working self-employed, we managed fairly well. I was, however, using my savings to keep us going and the money began to run out shortly before my major operation. I began to worry about how we were going to manage. I did, however, have wonderful support from my church. It offered to pay me the same rate as I'd been paid while working part-time for as long as it took to get me through surgery, the aftermath and back on my feet.

Following my operation I resumed work after three months. There were no benefits I was entitled to because I was earning above the threshold. It was at this time that my financial worries became acute, because by now all my savings had gone and after the bills had been paid there was very little left for anything else. In September 2001, however, I was offered a family support job at a local hospice. It involved pre- and post-bereavement counselling skills, for which I was fully qualified, as well as a good remuneration. This meant my financial worries considerably lessened

I had a number of issues relating to the stoma bag to deal with that I clearly had to sort out in my mind, to ensure that I didn't begin to lose the confidence that I so very much needed as an ostomist. You can suffer emotional distress when people know about your situation. For example, you may worry, as I did, about whether people can see the bag, whether it smells, what people are thinking or saying and the problems you will face when you grow older and find it difficult to cope. I found, however, that if I faced the problems with a positive attitude and carefully focused on them with the desire and determination to solve them, they were no longer so great and became surmountable. Sometimes the problem was not really a problem at all; it was simply something that I had created in my mind.

The answer to the question 'Can you see the bag?' is both yes and no. Yes of course it can be seen when you are undressed. But almost always the only people who will see you undressed are those you want to see you like this. In my opinion being seen by your loved ones in a state of undress with a stoma bag in place is a most positive step to recovery from the psychological effects of stoma surgery. If you let your spouse or others close to you see you naked with the stoma bag attached to the stoma you will have overcome a major hurdle as far as accepting yourself, and others accepting you, for what you are.

When you are fully clothed, however, the bag cannot be seen. Although you are obviously aware that it is there, others are oblivious to this fact. I wear a two-piece bag, a pouch that can be drained with a flange and a small belt that clips on to the appliance for added security. The flange is a round, moulded piece of flexi-soft plastic with a hole tailored to fit around my stoma. The side that fits to my body is highly adhesive and sticks like cement, providing a secure and watertight bond to my abdomen. This bond is actually strengthened by water so that when I have a bath or shower I feel totally secure.

The flange has a rim around the stoma and a stoma bag, with

the same-size hole as the stoma, is clipped on to the flange, providing a very secure and safe fitting. The bottom of the bag is folded around a plastic clip to seal it. This clip can be removed when the bag needs to be emptied. For added security I wear a very light belt that clips on to the bag. I wear the flange for four days and then discard it and replace it with a new one. The bond is so strong that the only way to remove it without ripping my skin is to use an adhesive remover.

The flange is very comfortable and discreet and usually I can't feel that I am wearing it at all. Over the stoma bag I wear the long, tight version of Lycra boxer shorts. For me they work very well and hold the bag flat against the stomach wall. You can't tell there is a bag fitted when I put them on and when I am fully dressed you can't see it at all.

I am very self-conscious and if I thought that there was any hint of my bag being seen by anyone I didn't want the bag to be seen by, I'd be horrified. But I know that only the wearer knows about the bag, or those whom the wearer chooses to show or tell. I do, however, speak openly about the bag. I have found that to casually mention my operation and the stoma and bag in a conversation with acquaintances, however embarrassing it might be at first, is better than not mentioning it and helps me to cope.

Does the bag smell? Yes, it does smell. There's no way around this. When you drain or change it, of course the bag smells, but no more than a visit to the toilet would smell.

Some people seem to have an in-built fear of people who have had a colostomy or ileostomy. They think they should give them a wide berth to avoid a dreadful odour. That, however, is very far from the truth. I thought like that myself before I had the operation. I didn't avoid people with stomas but often wondered if they smelt. I now know that there is no smell because the smell is contained within the bag.

Medical science has moved forward at a phenomenal pace and

those of us who have recently had major surgery have benefited from the new technology. Not that many years ago there were horror stories of people who had undergone permanent ileostomies and how they found great difficulties in coping with stoma bags. In 2006, however, these bags are far more user-friendly, wearable … and don't smell.

Diet plays a big part in preventing odour. I found I had to be careful to avoid or only ingest small amounts of food or spices that might increase the possibility of a smell. Experience plays a big part in this; no one wants to risk bad odours. You learn very fast about what not to consume.

As far as what people think or say is concerned, it is by far the best policy not to think or worry about this. Life is too short. Also, you don't know what goes on inside people's heads. You are probably worrying unnecessarily. It's a worry that you're creating; it's not a fact, it's a fictional worry. We spend so much time worrying about what other people might think or say about us. Unfortunately, we often allow our minds to battle with imaginary worries that result in nothing but pain and misery. We may let ourselves be wound up or intensely upset over something that might not have happened the way we have perceived it. Or there may have been something that we thought was being said about us when it was nothing of the sort. It is so easy to get wound up about something in particular and blow it up out of all proportion.

Over the years I have often been wrong about things that have happened. For example I once thought someone was talking about me because I saw this person huddled together with others looking my way. But I was wrong. I have been intensely anxious because of what I thought someone might have said or what he or she might think of a particular situation relating to me. But it was all conjecture. My thoughts were not related to what was actually happening.

We need to practice being realistic about our situation. Anxiety leads to misery and fear. I believe we need the peace of God. St

Paul in the Bible says: 'Be anxious for nothing, but in everything by prayer and supplication, with thanksgiving, let your requests be made known to God; and the peace of God, which surpasses all understanding, will guard your hearts and minds through Christ Jesus.' (Philippians 4:6-7).

At the end of the day what does it matter what people think? As an ostomist I know that what someone else thinks is not going to change my situation. People are people and, sadly perhaps, we form our own ideas about a particular scenario, whether right or wrong. An ileostomy or colostomy may be for life. Whether I'm happy or unhappy with the situation I'm in, unless a solution to the problem can be found as an ileostomist I'm stuck with it. I find it far better to accept my condition and get on with life rather than continually worry about what people think of me in my situation, and that is what I try to do with God's help. I believe that God offers peace. He can take the mindless anxiety away, but first I have to give the situation to Him and then try to get on with my life.

Another worry of mine was what I would do when I became old and found it difficult to cope. Although we have to think about what will happen when we get old and try to provide as much as possible in the way of financial security for this eventuality, I think it can be very unnecessary and unprofitable to worry about the future in any great detail. To be mindful of something by really facing up to what it means and being realistic about the possible outcome is sensible. Issues that happen, that crop up without warning, have to be faced and shouldn't be avoided. We have to deal with our responsibilities and not be in denial about matters we may not want to face up to. But to fret and worry about something to the extent that it begins to take over our everyday lives is extremely counter-productive. Worry is a waste of time and energy. Worry has been said to be like a rocking chair, it keeps you moving but takes you nowhere.

The issue of ageing and being unable to cope was one of the

first I began to think about when I realised that a permanent ileostomy was the only answer to the UC. At the time I knew I had a choice. I could constantly worry about the future and what would happen to me when I was in my eighties. Or I could get on with my life and learn to live one day at a time.

I realised that at fifty-four years old when I had the operation, God willing, I probably had a lot more living to do. If that were the case what good would it do to think about what might happen to me when I was older? The exercise would be pointless because I might not live that long, in which case I would have been worrying about the future for nothing.

Being a Christian is wonderful because I believe God has the answers to all things and that He will guide us on the way forward if we call out to Him. I believe He doesn't want us to worry about our lives and get stressed out so that we become frustrated and ill. Jesus said: 'Therefore do not worry about tomorrow, for tomorrow will worry about its own things. Sufficient for the day is its own trouble.' (Matthew 6:34).

Life can be so stressful. You only have to walk into a supermarket on a Saturday afternoon to discover this. Living our lives brings us choices, and we live our lives by the choices we make. Sometimes what happens is out of our control. Nevertheless there are many decisions an individual has to make that will affect the way he or she lives. In my opinion, looking far ahead and worrying about a situation that has not yet happened or might never happen is unwise. Taking one day at a time can be much less stressful. Most terminally ill people try to practise the art of living only one day at a time, as do recovering alcoholics. What they're faced with in any given day is possibly more than enough to cope with without added worries related to events in the future. I, too, have decided to try to live one day at a time. I've found it's something you have to discipline yourself to do; it's not necessarily easy to achieve and it needs a lot of work. I think though that the positive results of a more stress-free life far outweigh the effort required to achieve it. All this doesn't mean that I never plan ahead; I do, very often. There are many people who live haphazardly, never really making plans, and who act on impulse. I'm not suggesting that anybody should live like this; I certainly don't. What I do think, however, is that it is better to step back from pressures related to the future and try to take one step at a time.

Living with an ileostomy or colostomy is not ideal, but it can be managed. I did not choose to have UC, but I did choose to have a permanent ileostomy. In my view my choice has meant I now lead a far better life than I would have done had I not had the operation.

9

ACCEPTING THE CHANGES

At the end of the last chapter I said that living with an ileostomy is not ideal but that it is manageable. In this chapter I shall build on this statement, showing in more detail what that means.

Living with an ileostomy or colostomy requires resilience; a determination that whatever happens you'll manage. At times the problems arising from the condition can be extremely daunting and it requires patience and a sense of humour to help to get you through the day.

Having a stoma can be messy, as the bag needs to be drained. In my case, I put a small bag on in the morning to get me through the day, draining this whenever required, perhaps three or four times a day. Before I go to bed I change this for a larger bag to cope with the day's output. You don't have to do this but it appears to work for me. It's quite tricky at first to manage the changes or drain the bag as you never know when the stoma is going to work. It doesn't have any muscle and so cannot control the unpredictable and uncontrollable contractions of the gut. The stoma can catch you out when you're least expecting it, leaving a mess all over the place. But you will get used to it and after a while become proficient in dealing with it, I assure you. It's all a matter of practice.

You'll know when the bag needs emptying by just touching the site of the stoma through your clothes. It is always advisable not to let the bag get too full. It may be a recipe for disaster if left too long. It's better to be cautious and empty the appliance when you feel you need to. You'll get to know when with practice. The stoma, the artificial opening of the tube that has been brought to the abdominal surface, will need time to adjust to your body. Also, when you first have a stoma you may find yourself emptying the bag far too often as paranoia will almost certainly try to kick in. Please try not to panic.

In my opinion it is best, if possible, to change or drain the appliance in a bathroom over the toilet bowl, with a sink close by to wash your hands afterwards. If you follow my suggestions set out below you will almost certainly avoid a mess and unnecessary embarrassment.

I kneel on a spongy kneeler, placing a baby's care mat on the floor at the toilet bowl to drain the bag. This not only helps to keep me clean but also prevents me from hurting my kneecaps. I fill a plastic jug with fairly warm water and have a plastic syringe ready. This holds enough water to flush out the bag after draining. (You may be able to get hold of the syringes from your stoma nurse.)

You may not be able to kneel down but you must be able to position yourself over the toilet bowl – try crouching – to allow the contents of the bag to drain down the toilet.

This works fine at home where you're familiar with the environment and know where you've stored the equipment you need. When you go out, however, you'll have to take some supplies with you and check out the toilets that you might have to use. Be prepared for as many eventualities as possible.

I carry a man's shoulder bag. Inside the bag, I put a couple of spare stoma bags, together with some wipes, scented disposable bags, and clips, my syringe and a disabled toilet key. You can apply for a disabled toilet key from the Royal Association for Disability and Rehabilitation (RADAR). RADAR operates the National Toilet Key Scheme. At the time of writing this book the key costs around £3 - £5 and is worth every penny. (The address and details are in the Useful Information on page 152.)

For a small charge, RADAR will also provide you with a small booklet that lists all the disabled lavatories throughout the UK. With the RADAR key you can use one of these toilets, which is unlikely to have been vandalised, and be in total privacy. Compared to public lavatories disabled toilets are a luxury.

Outside the home toilets can be a great worry. You need to think carefully before you use one. For instance, there may be no toilet paper available and this can be a big problem when draining the bag. Make sure you carry some toilet paper in your kit; it can be a lifesaver. The floor may be wet, making kneeling impossible, so you will have to find some other way of positioning yourself over the toilet bowl. If it is not a disabled toilet there may be a big gap under the door and walls, offering no privacy. Also there may be no washing facilities or water available. You could carry a small bottle of water around with you or in my opinion better still, purchase a collapsible water bottle that you can fill from a tap prior to going into a cubicle. These are excellent as they fold up like a concertina and fit in your carry bag very easily. They can be found in any art shop at a very small price. Always try to find somewhere else if the toilet isn't suitable. Sometimes, though, this is just not possible and you may just have to grin and bear the embarrassment.

You have to adapt and be able to manage with the facilities and equipment available. This only comes with experience. Nevertheless with forward planning and the use of your initiative such problems can always be solved. If you have prepared beforehand and have your kit with you, you're more than half way there. And try as hard as you can not to panic. Panic won't get you anywhere.

There may be occasions when you go out and, even though you drain the appliance just before you leave home, find that it needs to be drained again as soon as you arrive at your destination. Try not to worry as this often happens. You'll get into a routine after a while but sometimes, even when you do so, the stoma may decide it's going to work. There may also be a rare occasion when the bag leaks when you're out. This can be distressing. Keep calm. Find a toilet, take your survival kit with you and slowly change the flange or the one-piece bag. Keeping calm can keep you going, panicking won't.

You have to make sure you have a continuous supply of bags and accessories. I use a delivery service as I find it very helpful. (See the Useful Information section on page 152.) The stoma nurse organised my first delivery and after that my GP gave me a repeat prescription. When I am getting low on supplies I tick my requirements on the prescription and take it to the surgery, where it will be dealt with within forty-eight hours. I then telephone my order and send my prescription through to the delivery service as soon as I receive it. The delivery service is very helpful and discreet in all it does. The people there know all the products and their serial numbers, whereas I've found chemists to be rather vague.

Although there needs to be some changes or adaptations to ensure your new life is fulfilling there is no reason why things have to change very drastically. You will still be able to take part in sports, including swimming, have sex, do gardening, drive, work, go to the pub, in fact do a host of things – although possibly not all at the same time. Joking aside, though, you do, of course, need to think carefully about how to plan the way forward in your new life and there is no reason why you shouldn't live a full life.

Since I've had my ileostomy I try to stay fit. Most evenings I go out for a vigorous walk. This is slightly less than two miles, but I do walk very fast. I find this keeps me in trim and helps to burn off the calories. I also do most things that I used to do in the garden before the operation. Hazel doesn't like me mowing the lawn. She tends to do this as she thinks I might damage my stoma if I move a heavy lawnmower about. I see her point and I'm careful. I usually do the trimming – but do occasionally set myself loose on the mower.

I've found I have to be careful about lifting heavy things. A year ago we purchased a large television, and I had to show that I was still a macho man by lifting it in and out of the car and then into the house. I subsequently spent a very agonising week with severe pains in my abdomen. I had not felt pain like this previously and my GP and stoma nurse showed little sympathy. It was a silly thing to do and I've learnt my lesson.

Once I'd recovered from the operation I wanted to resume sexual relations with Hazel. But having a bag stuck on to my abdomen didn't exactly make me feel I was a great catch. I worried about how Hazel would react to my advances. We had talked through the possible difficulties of resuming a sexual relationship prior to the operation, but talking is different to performing and I wasn't sure what would happen. I decided to roll the bag up and tape it to my abdomen so that it was out of the way. Although everything was strange initially our first sexual encounter after the operation went very well and Hazel responded to me as she had done previously. She did, however, say afterwards that she had been frightened she would hurt me.

The downside was when I had an orgasm. It felt different, almost as if nothing had really happened. We decided to leave it for a few days and then try again. This time I noticed I was not ejaculating. There was no semen and very little by way of a climax. I remembered that the doctors had told me that there was a risk of nerve damage with the type of surgery I'd had.

I saw a doctor and my surgeon shortly afterwards, and mentioned my experience. He told me it was something called retrograde ejaculation. With this condition it means that the semen is ejaculated backwards into the urinary bladder instead of out of the penis. It is probably caused by damage to the nerves as a result of surgery. I could get an erection but failed to have a proper orgasm, which was not only disappointing and frustrating but also worrying. My GP told me that with time the situation might improve, but he was extremely doubtful about this.

It has been six years ago, now, since I saw these medics. There has been a slight improvement. I still cannot ejaculate externally, but I do get some form of climax, although it's nothing like it used to be. This does bother me; I would be lying if I said it didn't. It has not, however, fundamentally changed our sex life. It has, though, played on my mind a bit and I've had to work hard to be positive about the situation.

Sex may be different but I have had to reassure myself that at least I can get an erection. We have sex when we want to. Admittedly it isn't as spontaneous as I would like it to be. I have to 'tape up', for one thing, and make sure my bag is empty before we begin, but it is still satisfying and Hazel and I are able to enjoy each other.

Whether you've had an ileostomy or colostomy your life will never be the same again, as you knew it before the operation. Ironically, though, for many the operation will be a blessing in disguise. As a UC sufferer, the disease seemed to run my life for me. I had to take endless amounts of various medications, including steroids, to manage each day. Now I don't take any medication. (Most ileostomists don't.) I've realised the ileostomy is permanent, that the stoma is for life and have decided that I might as well learn to live with it and try to enjoy it. It's much better than having UC or cancer.

There are people who have had to have either an ileostomy or colostomy forced upon them, sometimes without their knowledge. This may have been because of an external accident. One moment someone may have been leading a full, active and happy-go-lucky life, the next he or she wakes up in a hospital ward to find that an operation has taken place. At least I had time to prepare myself for my operation and all that it entailed. It must be awful to find out that suddenly you no longer function as you did previously, and extremely difficult to cope. But for those to whom this has happened I assure you that there is life out there. Go for it and don't give up. Your life may not be the way you planned it would be, but nevertheless you are living and life can be enjoyed.

A change in someone's life can be extremely stressful and difficult to manage. Some people manage major events in their lives relatively easily. For others changes cause major problems, ones they need help with. Changes happen throughout our lives. We are born, go to school, grow older, achieve, fail, fall in love, fall out of love and suffer bereavement. Change, however joyful, also brings loss. We fall in love and for a while leave our stable lives behind; we have children and lose sleep and time for ourselves. People come and go in our lives; jobs are found and sometimes lost; hopes may be shattered as loss inevitably brings about change that we hadn't bargained for. We are constantly faced with the need to give up one thing and accept another.

It is difficult to accept something that we have not chosen. We then need to look at the possible options. We can refuse to accept what has happened. This, however, will lead nowhere as we need to be able to cope with the reality of the situation. We can accept the situation grudgingly, but this way may well lead to bitterness and a constant moan of 'if only'. But we can also accept the situation as it is and learn something from both the situation and the acceptance. This will almost undoubtedly create a positive outlook on what has happened.

We never know what lies around the corner. We cannot be sure what is going to happen in the next minute, let alone the next hour. Life events come and go and it makes sense to make the attempt to get on with life, to go with the flow instead of constantly fighting against it. I am not saying that we should accept every situation that comes our way and become a doormat. Some things can and need to be challenged and resisted. Others, however, need to be accepted for what they are.

If we lived in a perfect world where nothing ever hurt us or damaged us in any way it would be wonderful. But we don't. We actually live in a world that can appear hostile at times and there are many times, perhaps all the time, when we may feel we are on our own. I believe that being a Christian is extremely comforting, because as a Christian you need never feel alone. But if you are a Christian is doesn't mean you won't suffer anything. The same rain that falls on the unrighteous also falls upon the righteous. Being a Christian does not mean that I'm exempt from experiencing all that happens in the world. If that were the case, I believe that Jesus would not have died the humiliating and horrific death that He did.

10

DARE TO ACCEPT – IT'S FOR LIFE

My purpose in writing this chapter has been to show the reader how my faith has helped me to stay sane and cope with UC and subsequent stoma surgery. The stresses and changes have been difficult to adjust to; if it had not been for my faith I think it would have been very much harder to deal with.

Hazel and I both feel we were not alone. Knowing God was there with us brought us comfort. We felt His presence gave us peace during the times when we needed it most. It is because of this that I felt the need to encourage you, whether or not you share my particular faith, that there is a way through.

As a professing Christian, after my operation I found that the rough had to be taken with the smooth and that exemptions from rough spells are not always available. Thus, although I'm a Christian, my Christianity didn't stop me from going through the ordeal of UC and stoma surgery. There were no special privileges because I was a believer. I realised it was essential to accept what had happened to me completely, so that I could understand and cope with my situation realistically and efficiently.

The acceptance, however, was very difficult to achieve. Even though I believed I had met with God in hospital and that He had given me the strength to make a rapid recovery, when I was discharged I felt very lethargic. My encounter with the

Almighty had been special. However, psychologically, I still had a long way to go.

I began to understand that a permanent ileostomy is a drastic and irreversible operation. The UC had robbed me of ten years of my life. I desperately wanted to feel better, to live my life without any further upheaval and heartache. But I was frightened to think that something might go wrong in the future. Fear seemed to dominate and I found this was difficult to control. I was, however, not afraid of dying. My faith was strong enough to help me believe that if I did die I would go straight to heaven. Nevertheless I didn't welcome the idea of dying at the time. I wanted to live and to live life to the full.

I began to experience the aftermath of the operation, which included weakness, pain and discomfort. In addition, I had to get used to a completely new lifestyle. But all this was no excuse for ignoring God. As a Christian I should have known better. I should have known that I needed Him more at this time than perhaps ever before. Having subsequently thought about my behaviour at this time, however, I think it was not a deliberate decision on my part to ignore God but more of a 'I can't be bothered' frame of mind.

Initially, once I got back home my spiritual situation could be described as hanging on by the skin of my teeth. Yet God had not moved away from me. He had not changed His mind about me or taken a holiday. It was just that I just couldn't feel Him. What is more I couldn't be bothered to seek His presence.

Within the first couple of weeks, however, I began to see that I needed to discipline myself to be able to move into God's presence. This meant spending time with God in prayer and reading the Bible. Christians believe that God is with us all the time and that He never leaves us. When, however, we are concentrating on Him through prayer, the feeling and awareness of Him is more intense. I believe you can feel His presence. In the Old Testament Jeremiah says 'Then you will call upon Me and go and pray to Me, and I will listen to you.

And you will seek Me and find Me, when you search for Me with all your heart.' (Jeremiah 29: 12-13). I had to be willing to surrender the way I felt by giving my fears and burdens to God and rely on His strength and guidance to help me through life. I had to give Him the first place in my life and call out to Him, knowing that He had the answers and the strength to help me through whatever situation I was in. At the time I knew that it was the last thing I wanted to think about or do. But I now know it was the most important.

God helps us to surmount obstacles that we are faced with, but not always in the way that we expect. For example when Daniel was in the lions' den, God didn't rescue him from certain death. Daniel still had to go through the ordeal of being in the den with the lions. But God sent angels to deliver him from the power of the lions surrounding him, keeping the lions still and their jaws closed. (Daniel 6: 10-23). The lions were there waiting for their next meal, but once God had intervened they had no power over Daniel. And in the face of adversity Daniel did not waver. He clung on to his faith in God and prayed three times a day, regardless of other people's threats. When he was in the lions' den it appears that he was still honouring God; he didn't appear to be resentful at all. He trusted his God (Daniel 6: 21-22). (He was not eaten by the lions but freed from the lions' den the following morning.)

I began to realise that sometimes we are not rescued from what we are going through. We are left wondering why and are not always given the answers. But I now believe that God knows best, even though I didn't think so at the time. I had to accept things I couldn't change instead of complaining and formulating other negative responses.

I could well have begun to feel sorry for myself and have acted in a childish manner because things were not going my way. But that type of behaviour serves no purpose. When I was a child I used to sulk if I couldn't get my own way. I would stick out my bottom lip and huff and puff. Inwardly I would seethe because things had not happened in the way I'd wanted them to happen. But this didn't change anything at all. I was acting like a spoilt child. My behaviour was not unusual. Many other people have behaved like this when they were children and unfortunately behave like this when they are adults as well. When other people's thoughts are contrary to some people's way of thinking and when things happen that are not what is wanted, pandemonium reigns. In bereavement work, for instance, patients or family members may well become angry because someone's terminal illness has been diagnosed. They may think that if only the doctor had acted sooner perhaps the illness would not have progressed so much. There is a refusal to accept the reality of what is happening and as a result there may be a breakdown in communication and trust between patient, family and medical staff. I have witnessed this many times in my career as a social worker and bereavement counsellor and during my years of pastoral counselling within the church movement. As adults we all behave like children at times, but as St Paul says, 'When I was a child, I spoke as a child, I understood as a child, I thought as a child; but when I became a man, I put away childish things' (1 Corinthians 13:11). As an adult childish behaviour serves no purpose.

As I began to focus on God, I began to remember how He had helped me so much in the past. He may not have given me all that I had asked him for and He may not have answered my prayers the way I had anticipated. Nevertheless I had felt that His love had always been around me and there were many times I remembered His rescuing power. I knew that there were many times I wouldn't have been able to manage if He had not been there to help me. I also remembered that the times I had received His help were the times that I had surrendered to Him. They were the times I was in touch with Him, calling to Him. He had been so faithful and I knew that He had been through every situation with me.

I have been a Christian for many years now and believe that with God's help I've been able to face many obstacles.

Sometimes I have wanted God to save me from an unpleasant situation, but God has not always answered my prayers. Also I now know He doesn't always answer my prayers the way I expect He should because He wants me to realise that 'My Grace is sufficient for you, for My strength is made perfect in weakness' (2 Corinthians 12:9). God's Grace helps me through very difficult and hard times. When I feel I have insufficient strength to manage, as I call upon Him He gives me the necessary strength. I believe that my Christian journey has shown me that His Grace is sufficient for anything that happens.

Some time ago something very bad threatened my professional career. Although I'd done nothing wrong, I couldn't deal with the problem, and this caused suffering for both my family and myself. I decided to ask God to help me. Because I called on God and gave him my problems, He demonstrated his power. When I told Him how weak I felt and that I was unable to solve my problem, He rescued me, but in a way I'd never contemplated. At the time He showed me He could give me all the peace that I needed.

I once again saw that God had a purpose for my life. I had foolishly forgotten that I knew about this before my operation. I learnt that in the midst of my pain and confusion God was with me. I realised I needed to keep focused on Him, otherwise I would become frustrated and lose sight of Him completely.

Both Hazel and I had been through years of my suffering UC. Then we struggled with the surgery and came through it together. There were changes that needed to be negotiated so that I could adjust to them. Nevertheless, they were negotiable and attainable. But I realised that I could only achieve my goal by asking for God's help. I couldn't achieve it on my own. I realised that He was my strength and that the only way I was going to manage was by praying to Him and asking for his help.

Gradually I began to focus on all that had happened to me

over the past few weeks. I thought about the way that God, rather than deserting me, had chosen to be right beside me through all my experiences. He had never left me and what is more I believed that He never would. That is because I believe He is committed to me. As the New Testament says, 'I will never leave you nor forsake you' (Hebrews 13:5).

I believe He is with us if we ask Him to be. No matter what we may go through He is never very far away. For some people like myself suffering can be extremely traumatic, leaving us with the thought that if He loves us, why does He allow so many bad things to happen? I do not know the answer to this, but my faith is strong enough to accept that God alone knows the answer.

I believe that God is the God of the Resurrection. He raises life out of death, good out of bad and growth out of pain. I do not believe that it is God's will or plan for anyone to suffer or be in pain forever. Even so I do believe that sometimes God intends us to go through suffering for a purpose. I may have suffered pain through UC and over the surgery period, but I'm in no pain now and in fact have never felt better. I believe God wants me to help others in the same or similar circumstances to my own and that in order to do so He wanted me to experience what others had or will suffer.

I have come to see that being a Christian may not change the situation that I'm in. My faith does, though, offer me someone who is prepared to share in whatever I'm going through. His Name is Jesus, the resurrected Son of God. I believe in Jesus and have known Him for twenty-six years. He has never let me down yet and I believe He never will. He might have healed me before I had to have surgery, but He didn't. Some people have asked me why. My reply is always the same. I say that Jesus is able to heal whomsoever He chooses, but that in my case he chose not to. I add that when I became a Christian I promised that I would do whatever He wanted me to do, would go wherever He wanted me to go and would say whatever He wanted me to say. In other words, I gave myself completely to Jesus.

I believe that God has never let me down. He could have healed the colitis, which would have meant I wouldn't have had to have the operation. But if that were the case I wouldn't be seeing and helping people who are having similar operations or who are in even worse circumstances that myself. How would I really have been able to understand what it is like to wear an appliance on a daily basis for life if I hadn't had the operation? I have no complaints about my present situation and I am very willing to serve God. I have hit rock bottom in my life and know what this feels like. But I have also felt Jesus lift me from rock bottom and put me back on my feet. This is because I believe He loves me.

I find acceptance to be extremely difficult to comply with. When things do not go my way and I'm forced to comply with what I'm faced with I'm tempted to think that I've failed. I'll do everything to believe what has happened is not what it appears to be. But when all else has been tried and when I've done all I know to change a given situation, and it still remains unchanged, I know that then is the time to think about whether what has happened is meant to be.

Acceptance is not a matter of giving up or throwing the towel in. We should never accept what has happened simply for the sake of a peaceful life. And some issues that crop up do need challenging. They conflict so much with our beliefs and values that it becomes impossible to accept what has happened. That is when you have to make a stand to bring about a more acceptable resolution to the circumstances.

As a Christian, I am called to be a person of faith, and I emphasise this. At times God's purpose is so clear that I have to accept what I'm going through, even though I don't like it at all. This is rather like Daniel's friends, Shadrach, Meshach and Abed-Nego, when they were faced with Nebuchadnezzar's image of gold (Daniel 3:1). In this instance, Nebuchadnezzar ordered everyone to worship a gold image. These three young men, however, refused to bow down to anyone except God and as a result were thrown into a fiery furnace. They could have accepted the situation that was being forced on them, but they made a stand against what they considered an evil declaration and had to accept the consequences of their action. They could do nothing else. They had done all they could. All that was left was to accept.

I, too, had to take a stand. I could well have given up on my faith. I was not being healed, the UC was devastating my life and the prospect of stoma surgery was extremely daunting. I had to make a decision to either face up to the reality of the situation, accept it for what it was and get on with my life, or give up. I felt I had to make a stand and that whatever I had to face I would face it head on, with my God at my side.

I think that learning to grow through the pain I've experienced has brought me great benefit. By this I mean that looking at and evaluating the reality of my situation, as well as re-channelling my thoughts more positively, has brought great comfort not only to my family and myself but also to other people who are in a similar situation to myself. If I had remained sorry for myself and had not had the operation, there would definitely not have been any room for growth in my life.

The Special Air Service (SAS) proudly and courageously bears the motto 'Who Dares Wins'. This statement means that whatever situation you may find yourself in you should deal with it, and that if you do you will achieve what you want. Never daring to run will not win races, and I think as an ostomist that there is a race to be run, that is, a life to be lived.

The Bible says 'I can do all things through Christ who strengthens me' (Philippians 4:13). As a Christian I can dare to do things through Jesus. I want to encourage you, whether or not you consider yourself to be a Christian, to dare to be different. Dare to live a life that will pave a way for others to benefit. You may have had surgery. You may not have coped very well with it up until now – I didn't myself. But pick yourself up and dare to start again. You can do it. Dare to believe that there is life out there and that life is for you.

Hazel and I do not know where we would be today if we did not believe that Jesus had helped us. I had no fight left in me when I was in hospital. I was weak and lethargic, frightened and apprehensive, but I believe that Jesus came to my rescue. It is true that I have fluctuated in my faith. I'm only human. But I believe that God understands this. It can also be said that wearing a bag is not ideal or that having a sexual dysfunction is hardly indicative of a loving God. I offer nothing in defence. I do have these disabilities. Nevertheless I have life and I believe that God who visited me in hospital has given me something to live for, and I shall never stop singing His praises. He has given me back my life and I will live it for Him.

He can do it for you too. He can change your life and give you the courage to go on, no matter what is ahead. Why not ask Him to help you?

If you have never asked Him into your life you can do it now by saying this prayer:

"Lord Jesus, I have lived my life for myself for too long. I now turn to You and ask You to help me. I ask You to forgive the sin that I have committed. I am sorry Lord, please live in my heart and be my Lord and Saviour and fill me with Your Spirit. I ask in Jesus' name. Amen"

You now belong to Jesus. Dare to believe it and get on with the life that He has planned for you. Get yourself a bible, an easy to understand version in everyday language; they are widely available from bookshops and churches. Join a lively and Spirit-filled church. Get baptised or immersed in water and live your newly found life with joy and excitement. Your life may not have gone the way you planned. It seldom does. But you have someone to share it with now – Jesus. Enjoy Him and let Him help you to find the purpose and destiny He has for your life. It has only just begun, whatever age you are! There is no ageism or redundancy, or retirement in the Kingdom of God.

11

WHERE'S THE CARER'S SUPPORT?

Hazel Howard

Grahame and I met in 1977 and got married in 1979. We have two daughters and a son, as well as five grandchildren.

In 1990 Grahame started to have frequent diarrhoea and pains in the stomach that didn't subside after the usual 'over the counter' remedies. After much persuasion he eventually went to see our GP who at first didn't think that Grahame had UC. Eventually, however, he referred Grahame to a hospital where UC was diagnosed and the first of many steroid medications was prescribed. There were many side effects of the pills and I think he became quite volatile in temperament, as a result of both the medication and the UC.

Slowly but surely Gray's illness began to take over not only his life but mine too. We could no longer have family or friends come to our home because of Grahame's constant fear of not managing to get to the toilet in time, or other people being in there when he needed it to be free for his use.

On Gray's fiftieth birthday we had sat and planned our future, including retirement, over a pub lunch. Four years' later in 1998 he had been ill-health retired and was about to undergo major surgery.

When Gray was retired, I was outwardly calm and supportive but inwardly devastated. Gray had worked so hard at university in 1993, studying for a Diploma in Social Work and Higher Education, and I had spent every night for two years on my own so that he could study. He passed his exams, obtained very good grades, then qualified as a social worker and got a good job. But here we were having lost all of this and left with nothing, without a future. Our plans were demolished, or so it seemed. I felt very disappointed and devastated; it seemed such a waste.

A social life was no longer possible and we couldn't do things together any more. UC had got such a hold on Gray by this time, and he was going to the toilet so frequently that going out was no longer a viable option. We would get in the car to go somewhere, but after ten minutes' drive down the road Gray would need to 'go'. Once we drove eight miles to our nearest town to do a bit of Christmas shopping, but as soon as we walked into a store Gray had an 'emergency'. He couldn't get to the nearest lavatory and there weren't any loos in the store that were available. As a result we ended up in an extremely embarrassing and degrading predicament. Of course, we had to get him straight back home and after a few occasions like that one he stopped going out.

Even so, we were able to talk together about what was happening and share things, and were also able to laugh together.

As Gray's carer there were some things that I felt and thought that wouldn't have been helpful or useful for him to know, such as my fear for him. So I talked to God about my worries and knew that my God would hear me, understand me and help me through.

When Gray had accidents, even in the house he wouldn't let me help him clear up the mess. He was so embarrassed, but all his embarrassment did was to frustrate me. (He was so poorly in the end, however, that he had no choice but to let me help him.)

We found it was essential to keep our sense of humour, and be able to laugh at things and with each other. One night lying in bed we talked about a name for Gray's bag when it had been fitted. After various suggestions he decided that that he was going to name it after his surgeon. The name has stuck and close family and friends are sometimes told 'Gray's in a meeting with 'Mr Rogers'. They know he's in the toilet draining the stoma bag, which can take about ten minutes. Occasionally we tell Mr Rogers to be quiet. This is because when the stoma begins to work it sometimes emits a burping or popping sound that can be quite loud.

When Gray had his colonoscopy he was still only half-conscious when he came back on the ward. He was not making a lot of sense. Then all of a sudden he started to sing at the top of his voice, 'Saved by the bell!' a line from a song by the Bee Gees. He never sang the rest of it, just that one line, and then went back to sleep. A little later he awoke and was more coherent, but didn't remember singing 'Saved by the bell' at all.

Gray was propped up on pillows and given a cup of tea, which he greatly relished. He had to wait to be discharged and so went to the lavatory. He seemed to be ages. I was getting a little concerned when the surgeon appeared and wanted to see Gray. He went off to see another patient so I went to fetch Gray out of the lavatory. But he couldn't find the lock on the door. He had become disorientated. He was on one side of the door laughing and I was on the other side also laughing. Fortunately he eventually managed to unlock the door and come out.

Having spoken to the surgeon he was discharged and allowed to go home. He had to get dressed, though. Gray being Gray, he insisted on doing this by himself. He tried to put one of his trainers on, slipped off the bed and banged his head on the wall. He then slumped on the floor. We both had hysterical giggles. It's a wonder we weren't thrown out of the hospital. I do think that a sense of humour and being able to really laugh can help to solve problems better than almost anything else.

When the medical specialist mentioned an operation to help Gray I had mixed emotions. I felt fear, shock, panic, but also a deep sense of relief. At last, after a very long time, it seemed that someone was actually going to do something other than give him yet another prescription. When we saw and spoke to the surgeon, however, we had a shock as he decided on a much more serious operation than either of us had anticipated. We had originally been told that Gray was going to have a colostomy as a temporary measure, to give his bowel some respite. The ileostomy, however, was a much more serious operation and, on this occasion, permanent. I was too shocked at the time to take in very much about what the man was saying.

We met the stoma care nurses who I thought were brilliant for Gray and came home with a bit more information. There was also a bag to look at if we wanted to, when we were ready for it.

It seemed there was this great big mountain in front of us, and that we had to climb it and get to the top before we could come down the other side. It seemed so impossibly big to me at the time. Even so I knew it had to be climbed. Sometimes I wasn't sure how we were going to do this, but deep down I knew that together we would manage. We had no other choice.

While we waited for the hospital date two men came to see Gray to talk about their operations. I really hoped they would bring their wives so that I could talk to their carers, but they didn't. I badly needed to talk to somebody who knew what I wanted to know, who had known what it was like to live with someone who had had UC, who had then had the operation to remove the disease, who could tell me about all the problems this might entail. I needed to talk to someone who knew what I was going through and the problems I was trying to face up to, as well as my thoughts, and could just be at the end of a telephone for me when I couldn't cope. But there wasn't anyone like that.

I did speak to one of the stoma nurses about my need to talk to other carers and asked her to give my telephone number to other carers if they wanted it, but I heard no more. I was scared, lonely, isolated, alienated from other people I knew who were not going through what I was going through with Gray, and I needed a friend.

As big as the mountain seemed, and as scared and lonely as I was, I knew that the God I had trusted in for the last twenty years or so would not let me down now. I knew I could stand on the promise of His words in Hebrews, 'I will not fail you nor forsake you' (Hebrews 13:5), and that He would be with me through it all because 'He who has promised is faithful' (Hebrews 10:23).

What we had to face up to was going to change our lives and we had to go through it, both together and yet each on our own. We considered the options of the permanent ileostomy and ileo-anal pouch very carefully, read and re-read the leaflets and books, and did eventually look at the bag. I offered my thoughts and opinions, which were that at our age and time of life, with Gray having had UC for such a long time, if he was going to go through surgery he might just as well go for the operation that was going to be successful from the outset, that is, the permanent ileostomy. This was so we could get the operation over and done with, and get on with our lives. Nevertheless, however, I knew and accepted that at the end of the day it was Gray and Gray alone who had to make the decision about what operation he was going to have.

My life was being dictated by Gray's illness. At times I just had to get out and away from it all, just for an hour for respite. I would go shopping or to a prayer group. I even went down to sit on the beach a couple of times, about two miles from our house. I needed to sit by the sea, breathe some air and think. Doing this gave me a feeling of space and a sense of living a normal life, even if only very briefly.

My sister and brother-in-law in Cambridge were celebrating their twenty-fifth wedding anniversary and were also re-taking their vows. I had been maid of honour at their wedding and it was really important for my sister and I to be together. But Gray was too ill for me to leave him and go to Cambridge on my own. I really resented this and had to struggle to keep control of my upset and disappointment. I was cross and angry because I couldn't go to where I wanted to go. It sounds a bit selfish now. But I resented Gray's illness and didn't see why it should interfere with as well as dictate my life. After all, it was his illness, not mine. I had to remind myself very firmly that it was not Gray's fault.

Preparations had to be made for Gray going into hospital for his major operation, such as buying him new pyjamas and a wash bag. So I kept us both busy with very short shopping trips. One day we bought a pair of slippers and a couple of days later a toilet bag. The preparations took ages.

I would sooner have driven Gray anywhere other than to the hospital, which was eight miles from where we lived. Eventually Gray was settled in the ward and things started to happen with the nurses tooing and froing, so I returned home. It was awful to leave him. He looked so scared and lost and alone. I felt totally helpless. There was nothing more I could do for Gray. I didn't want to leave him alone in a strange environment with strangers to look after him. I had a fear of the unknown and what was going to happen and was aware that the next time I would see him the operation would have been done. I didn't know what that was going to be like for either of us. He was going to be operated on the following morning.

We had our little dog Chips at home, my constant companion, comfort and friend. I had to come home to feed him, walk him and care for him. He loved being cuddled and in cuddling him I found some comfort. If we hadn't had a dog I would have stayed at the hospital all the time.

Having not slept much, by 8.30 the following morning, while Gray was being taken into theatre, Chips and I started to paint the kitchen woodwork. I am the type of person who has to work when stressed. If I'm upset or otherwise anxious I will throw myself into anything that totally absorbs me, both mentally and physically. Chips died in June 2004. I spent every day for three weeks in the garden digging up a tree that had died and then filled the hole back in again. Weird? Maybe. But that's me for you.

I phoned Gray's ward at 1 p.m., which is what I'd been told to do. Gray wasn't there. I was told he was probably in the recovery room and to phone back at 2 p.m. I had lunch and phoned again at 2 p.m., but he was still not back on the ward. The nurse then said, 'In fact, I don't know where he is. I'll find out though, and phone you straight back, I promise.'

'What?' I replied. 'Where is he? What's happening? Is he all right?' I was panicking and felt a terrible anxiety and fear. My heart started racing although I tried to keep calm. But the staff nurse was as good as her word and did phone me back to tell me to make my way over to the hospital as she'd found out that Gray was about to come out of the recovery ward.

When I arrived at the hospital I was very shocked. I hadn't known what to expect at all. No one had told me how he would be the first time I saw him. The specialist nurse who was settling him and checking the drips and monitors spoke to me briefly outside his door to let me know that the operation had gone well but that he was rather drowsy at the moment. Gray was in a side room by himself. There were drips, leads and tubes everywhere. He had lost so much weight, just overnight, and looked like a very sick, little old man. He opened his eyes momentarily, saw me and started to cry. I just held him and kissed his head. I couldn't let him see my emotions. Having hidden my feelings and emotions for a very long time, I had become a dab hand at appearing to be calm and collected when asked, and would say that I was all right when I really wasn't. Thus when the specialist nurse asked me how I was I said 'Fine, thank you'. I sat on the chair next to his bed and read a book while he drifted in and out of sleep. The specialist nurse was in and out of the room all the time, checking on him.

The staff at the hospital looked after Gray really well. There were fearful times when he started to be sick and his temperature and blood pressure were so erratic, but everyone was very attentive. The time of waiting for the test results to come back was also very difficult. But I felt that at this time God led me to a passage in the Bible. It was the second half of Isaiah 38:21. It says 'And he shall recover...'. That was all I needed. A specific word from God to keep me from fear. I believed that because of my faith in God, whether or not Gray had cancer, he would recover. The tests came back. There was plenty of colitis but no cancer. My prayers had been answered.

There came a day when the stoma nurse told me that Gray was ready for me to see the stoma. I was also ready for this. I had thought it through and Gray and I had discussed the issues about it together before the operation. Even so, when I first saw it I just cried, saying, 'What have they done to you?' I hadn't really known what to expect. Even so the stoma didn't upset me that much. It reminded me of a very large belly button. It was relatively easy for me to accept as I'd already seen my mother having her dressings changed following a mastectomy. The stoma was nothing in comparison to that.

After a while Gray began to get stronger and stated putting pressure on the hospital staff for him to go home. I, however, was not ready for this and kept trying to talk him into waiting awhile, pleading with him that he should patiently stay in hospital for as long as the medical team thought he should. But he insisted on going home. I was really frightened. What if we couldn't cope? What if he couldn't manage? What if I couldn't manage? We didn't know what Gray's coming home was going to mean for us as far as problems were concerned.

Just before Grahame came home, I got back from the hospital in the evening tired and hungry. By the time I sat down to eat a microwave meal it was nearly 10 p.m. I started to eat and burnt my mouth, as the food was so hot. I suddenly lost control, threw a fork at the wall and screamed my head off. It scared my little dog to death. Goodness knows what the neighbours thought. It relieved some of the pressures and afterwards I didn't feel quite so stressed. But I didn't cry, though I've shed many tears whilst writing this as I have re-lived the memories. I've realised that I didn't cry very much at all when Gray had his major operation. There were a few times when I shed silent tears, but I never had a really good cry. Maybe the tears that are falling now are the tears I should have shed then.

Gray got his way and I brought him home earlier than had originally been planned. He was so thin and very tired. He had to eat lots of tiny meals. At first just getting up from the chair he was in exhausted him and most nights he was in bed by 6 p.m. There were many little things he couldn't do initially, such as put on his socks, shoes or even trousers.

I once more became very fearful. I couldn't and wouldn't leave him on his own. Initially I'd only leave the room if he was settled in a chair and then I'd only go as far as the kitchen or bathroom. If friends came to the house to visit Gray I'd go off shopping for half an hour or so. At mealtimes I was a constant nag, reminding Gray of the eating rules: *small mouthfuls, put your fork down, sit back, chew your food, do not talk, eat slower.* Whenever he went to the toilet he obviously wanted his privacy, but I begged and made him promise not to bolt the door, just in case. At night I was scared stiff in case I hurt him in my sleep. So I put a pillow between us to prevent me knocking him.

I desperately wanted him to show me how to look after his stoma in case there ever came a time when he couldn't do this himself. But he was not ready to show me. I had to wait a long time. Only recently, four years later, has he shown me how to do this.

The stoma care nurses and district nurses came to visit frequently at first, which was good for me as well as for Gray because I saw someone else for a change, even if only briefly. Slowly but surely, day by day, Gray grew stronger and started to be a little more independent. Little by little we began to pick up the threads of a normal life. The problem was, though, Gray thought he could do more than he actually could, simply because he felt better. I had to make him really think for himself before he went off to do the garden or drive the car. I had to be very careful not to be too bossy. At the same time I had to try not to be too over-protective and to allow him to try to do things.

We had been given a dietary leaflet with brief information about foods and their possible effects, and what to avoid. As Gray's appetite increased, he ate a little of everything, and if he didn't have a problem with what he ate, he kept that food in his diet. The only foods he found he couldn't digest were celery and sweet corn. He now eats and drinks everything else without any problem. I do, however, reckon that beer and lager inflate 'Mr Rogers' fast if drunk quickly. This is because fizzy drinks cause excessive wind that tends to inflate the bag.

I've found the stoma bag is not a problem for me. Of course I would have preferred Gray not to have needed it. But the stoma has enabled us to have a better quality of life than when Gray was ill with UC. We both agree that we have got our lives back since the operation. Nothing can really prepare you for it though.

I do think carers need greater support. There needs to be someone working with stoma nurses who can provide support to carers, who need a listener and a confidante, a befriender, supporter and advisor who will reassure and empathise with them, and be easily contactable. More than anything carers need a personal point of contact and support, a one-to-one back up.

Life is very much better than it was six years' ago, for both of us. We have found that it is good to push boundaries to see what and how much Gray can do. (I'm aiming to get him on an aeroplane, but as yet we haven't quite got that far, although we do plan to visit Australia in 2007.) Gray has to experiment with new ways of doing things, all the time being aware of how he can cope with 'Mr Rogers'. Together we set goals and push boundaries and when Gray is ready we go for it.

Our sex life has, of course, been affected. I have had to reassure Gray constantly that he doesn't turn me off. We have been through a few ups and downs and it is taking time to re-establish a good sexual relationship, but we continue to work things through. At first my greatest worry was that I might hurt Gray, but that worry has now faded. We have both ended up quite frustrated at times, not only sexually but also emotionally with each of us blaming ourselves for whatever problem there might be. But in fact neither of us need to blame ourselves.

Grahame's determination over the years has at times been the one thing that has kept us going. He lives life in the fast lane. A GP once told me not even to try to keep up with him because, he said, I wouldn't be able to and that he'd only wear me out. He is also a very sensitive person and can get hurt quite easily, but tends to bounce back again just as quickly. He's quite impatient. He's working on that at the moment. I reckon that on the day of his funeral he'll be in the ground with his headstone in place before the rest of us have even got into our cars.

We have had the added difficulty of my going through the menopause these past few years. With me suffering from low libido, increasing hot flushes and mood swings, all this hasn't helped to make things easier in the bedroom. Nevertheless one recent discovery is that we can still be sexually spontaneous to a certain degree, which is very good news. This may be because our fears are lessening, or perhaps we are just getting more adventurous. (Since the operation until recently, quite a lot of planning ahead has been required – as though we had to book an appointment for sex.)

To cope with Gray's illness, operation and subsequent life we've had to work through problems together. We've had to talk at lot, make sure we don't blame either one another or ourselves and be honest with each other. Most important of all is that I've found I constantly need to reassure Gray that he is still as attractive to me as he's ever been.

I hope that what I've said will help other carers. Please remember that you are not alone. If you want to contact me, my email address is listed in the 'Useful Information' section on page 151 at the end of the book.

12

WAS IT ALL WORTH IT?

I cannot emphasise enough how much the operation has changed my life for the better. Before I went into hospital everything was bleak. I was ill, often in pain and had to take large doses of pills. If we had friends round for a meal they would have to be told about my condition so that they understood why I made so many visits to the toilet.

Although this was embarrassing, it was far better to have a meal in our own home than suffer the far worse humiliation of having a meal at someone else's. On arrival, I would immediately have needed to find out where the lavatory was. I would also have had to make sure I could have made it in time if I'd needed to go – which was inevitable – and would have had to have given a full explanation of why this was necessary to my hosts. My behaviour, needless to say, did nothing to help build relationships.

Furthermore, at home I 'owned' the toilet and to a degree could dictate its use in a most possessive manner. Using someone else's toilet, however, meant I had to forfeit ownership; I couldn't have control over the room. This may sound strange, even arrogant perhaps, to anyone who doesn't suffer from UC, Crohn's Disease or other serious bowel conditions, but it is something that IBD sufferers would understand.

Hazel's sister lives in Cambridgeshire and any free time we have we like to spend visiting her. We make this a holiday. But even making this visit became problematic because of the UC. Would I manage the journey without having an accident? When we arrived would the toilet be free? (They have a large family.) Would I be a nuisance? All this would mean I would become very anxious and stressed, and it would make Hazel and I wonder if it was worth the visit.

It would have been impossible to visit a restaurant, no matter what the occasion. The colitis could strike at the most inconvenient times. Not only would it have been a complete waste of money, but also would have meant the evening would have been ruined, and possibly Hazel in tears.

Even a simple and formerly enjoyable exercise such as shopping had become a nightmare. I would get inside a store and suddenly realise that I immediately had to get to a loo. Very probably the store would not have a public toilet and I had to suffer the indignity of having an accident right where I was. Of course that was the end of the shopping trip, and it was back home to change and miss out on what everyone else took for granted. It was easier not to go anywhere and I became a prisoner in my own home. As Hazel did not usually want to be on her own outside the house, it meant that she also quite often became marooned at home with me in my sorry state.

Yes, I can now hold my hands up high and shout that I'm very pleased that I've had the operation. I have my life back again. I'm now free from the clutches of UC. I'm free from having to take medication on a daily basis; in fact I now don't have to take any at all. I feel so much stronger and full of energy and vitality. It is a great pleasure to be able to walk over the fields or along the beach without getting caught short like I used to when I had UC. I have a new-found freedom, a freedom that I have not had for years and I'm still discovering what I can do with it.

I like to go bird watching and walk around the countryside. Whereas this was out of the question previously, it has now become eminently feasible and I feel like a child with a new toy. I am so grateful I have my life back. I don't know how long I could have gone on being like I was. I had nothing to offer anyone. I had lost my job and career through the illness and had really very few prospects. I am also so grateful to Hazel that she stayed with me and was my constant friend, supporter and confidante, and I'm grateful to God for giving her to me.

Men can be so vain and I'm no exception. Before my operation, and perhaps following a shower or getting dressed in the morning, I would often look in our full-length mirror in the bedroom at my naked or partly clad body and think to myself: just look at that! Not bad for a man of my age. I would stick out my chest and hold my stomach in like a not quite Mr Universe while I relished the sights that only I could see. But the first thing I noticed after my operation was the bag that sits on the right hand side of my abdomen. Somehow my dashing physique didn't quite look the same. The illusion was gone and I had to settle for the reality of what I looked like.

It took a while to get used to the changes and what I had become, but like all things associated with the ileostomy I have accepted the reality of my condition. With each problematic issue, I have thought about it, looked at it from a more positive perspective and have gradually learned to accept it. Thus I may never appear in *Playgirl* magazine as a nude male model, but then again I never wanted to in the first place. So I've not lost anything.

I've found that since the operation underwear has to be chosen carefully. Before surgery I would wear very small briefs that helped to enhance the male form. I now have to be mindful of the fact that I have a stoma and that attached to this is a stoma bag. Briefs are therefore not possible because the bag would just hang down underneath them, thus totally spoiling any illusion I might still have about my figure. What I have found is that tight-fitting boxer shorts are excellent and hide the bag perfectly. These are not only comfortable and secure but also boost my confidence as they are really quite presentable.

It helps that I'm married to a very understanding and supportive wife. She keeps my feet on the ground and reassures me when necessary. If I didn't have her, however, I think I would still take a positive approach to living. I have realised that being an ostomist is for life and that I need to accept my situation and live with it. I have no other choice. When things go wrong in our lives and we are knocked to the ground we can either lie there (and, let's face it, it's pleasant to do so at times) or we can get back up and look for a way forward. I chose the latter. I think we have to fight to live a life worth living or we'll never make it.

In the later stages of my UC I ballooned in size because of the steroid treatment and found I couldn't get into many of my clothes. I had to buy new clothes in a larger size. I kept the old clothes for the time when, following a strict diet, I would once again fit into them. That time never came, alas. I tried in vain to lose weight, but with the medication I was taking I was fighting a losing battle.

Exercise such as jogging or walking wasn't possible, as I was frightened I might get caught short and have an accident whilst I was out. Ordinarily, going to the toilet very frequently would have helped to keep me slim. Sadly, though, the steroid treatment caused the weight gain.

After the operation, however, I found that I'd lost a tremendous amount of weight and that my new clothes no longer fitted me. In fact one morning I put on a pair of trousers and they fell down to my ankles, even with a belt on. It was good, therefore, that I'd saved some of my old clothes. They fitted, although they were a little loose at first.

Most people make plans. Plans for future events such as

holidays, marriages, moving house, retirement, etc. Some people plan the day ahead; in other words they have an agenda. UC sufferers have to plan as well. If they suffer badly with the disease they have to plan any expedition they make outside the home around available lavatories. It is essential to know where the conveniences are for emergencies, and it's when you get to this stage that UC starts to rule your life.

But now I don't have to worry about this any more and it's marvellous. The fear of being in a public place and suffering the humiliation of soiling myself has now gone. There is a slight risk that the flange might spring a leak or that the bag might come off, but that's highly unlikely. It's true that ostomists need to make preparations for a day out, but not in the same great detail that they had to before they had the operation, that is, assuming they suffered from a serious bowel disorder. All you have to remember is that the bag will need draining or changing at some point during the day, and that you have the necessary resources available to meet this need.

Little by little, my confidence has returned, but it has taken a long time to do so. I have had to climb a mountain that at times I've not felt like climbing. Sometimes I've felt that what has happened has been so unfair. But I've also felt humbled having seen many people who are terminally ill who would give anything to have a longer life, even give up their gut and live with a stoma. I realise that I'm fortunate and have a life, and that my life is for living. I intend to make the best of what I've got, and that's a lot.

There is a new trend for disabled toilets to be shared with mothers who need to change their babies' nappies. I'm concerned about this because this trend is unfortunately disadvantageous to disabled people. Disabled toilets are especially equipped for disabled people. The money-saving device of allowing another use for disabled toilets limits their use for people with disabilities.

People with stomas cannot go into an ordinary toilet and use the facilities like other people, not without it being problematic at times. The bag may need draining or perhaps changing, or perhaps the flange may need some attention. A syringe may be required to flush the bag out, and then hands need to be washed before you can rearrange your clothing. All this takes time, and special toilets with special facilities are required. There is also an additional problem. I have often used a disabled toilet and have been in the middle of dealing with my appliance when someone has suddenly banged on the door. This may be because he or she thinks the room has been engaged for some time and for too long. Or it may be because it is thought there is someone locked in the toilet who has been taken ill. I have also had to suffer indignant looks from mothers when at last I come out of the toilet and they see that I've neither a noticeable disability nor a child with me. This causes me embarrassment and stress. It shouldn't be like this.

Most things you want to do will need a bit of planning from the moment you have recovered from your operation. You will need to think through things. Even travelling on a train will be a challenge. Changing or draining an appliance on a fast-moving train is an unforgettable experience and not one for the fainthearted. Nevertheless it will give you a great thrill to overcome something that you thought would be impossible.

Having a travel certificate can help you to travel abroad. This certificate is validated by your GP and explains what the appliances are for and that metal parts may be used and should be checked only in the presence of a medical practitioner. The certificates are in a number of languages and may help to avoid many embarrassing questions. You can obtain this from an ostomy association such as the National Office, or stoma care manufacturers such as ConvaTec. If you are an ileostomist you could join the IA, which is a national support association with local groups in your area. For a small annual fee the support is extremely good. For the colostomist there is the British Colostomy Association that provides equally good service and would also be able to advise on a travel certificate. For information about all these organisations see the 'Useful Information' list on page 151.

If you go to a hot country, pouches can be kept cool by putting them in a dry receptacle and placing them in a refrigerator. A first-aid kit is also wise. This should contain anti-diarrhoea treatment and fluid replacement powder. The ostomist should take special care abroad as it is so easy to become dehydrated. It is a good idea to talk to a stoma care nurse before travelling.

Some airlines will provide a seat near a toilet if you explain your situation when you book. If you are booking online, however, you may not be able to do this. It would in any case be better to contact someone on the phone to explain your needs. Airlines might also allow an extra luggage allowance for medical supplies. Don't forget to carry some spare kit in your hand luggage.

If you are reading this while waiting to go into hospital for an operation, please be reassured that life *will* get better for you. It will not be easy, but you will not have to manage alone. You will be well supported and nursed whilst in hospital, and you will not be allowed home until the doctors are satisfied that you will be able to manage. The final outcome, however, very much depends on you and your attitude towards your future life. You and nobody else are the one who has to live your life and it is surely best if you work very hard to try to live life to the full.

If you have suffered for any length of time with a serious bowel disorder, an operation for a stoma may have to be the only way forward, frightening though this may seem. If this is so try to focus on all of the positive aspects of your life after surgery. The nursing staff and doctors will have told you it is for the best and that you will feel much better. I was initially sceptical when I was told this, because after all I was the one who was going to have to go through with the operation, not them. I realise now, however, that it's true. The operation is painful but bearable, and someone is always on hand to alleviate the pain as soon as possible. You will feel very weak. Before the operation I hadn't thought about how weak I would feel. When I'd had it I felt at first as though I'd been run over by a large truck and I felt lifeless. You may feel the same. It will probably take all of your strength just to sit up and get out of bed, but each day you will get stronger. Within a couple of weeks you will be moving about and will soon return home.

After the operation you'll be very thirsty, but you won't be allowed to drink anything. The nurses will probably give you something to wash and wet your mouth with, but don't be tempted to swallow the liquid. After a day or two you may be put on 'Sips' and this is when you'll need to take it very easy. Don't do what I did and gulp the water. You will have had major surgery and your stomach will have been invaded and battered around. It will be very tender for quite a while, so you'll need to treat your physical self with as much tenderness as you would wish others to treat your mental self. If you try to gulp the water down before your stomach is ready, your stomach will repay you by ejecting it and you'll feel awful. I know this as this happened to me and I paid the price for my foolishness.

When you return home, usually within a two-week period, you will soon be getting on with your life again. But don't try to rush the convalescence period. Read that book you've been promising yourself to read and don't try to do too much too fast.

I thought I'd be trapped forever with UC. I couldn't see a way through. Now, however, I can honestly say that I'm glad to be an ileostomist. I can do far more than I could before. I'm working again full time in a local hospice as a bereavement counsellor. The work is very demanding but rewarding. I never thought this would be possible when I had to retire because of my ill health.

To summarise what I've already said in this chapter: I no longer have UC; I'm no longer on any medication; I'm no longer in pain; I can move around freely; I love the freedom; I've got my life back again; and I'm living it to the full. Truly the operation was very much worth it.

13

COUNSELLING AND ALTERNATIVE THERAPIES

Throughout this book, I have discussed my Christian beliefs in a lot of detail. What I believe in has been paramount in helping me to cope and find a way through the trauma and devastation that I found myself in whilst I had UC. Christianity gives me the strength and encouragement to face each and every day. It is, of course, not a remedy or a cure but a complete way of life.

Very soon after I got back from hospital after my surgery, when I was able to get round a little, I found that I got a great deal of satisfaction by just strolling around the woods and fields near my home. It was sheer bliss to walk in the woods and, for the first time in my life, to pick up a leaf and study it in detail, or simply to observe the birds as they busied themselves with gathering food. Just being able to have the time to commune with nature was so relaxing and satisfying. I am convinced that I was able to burn off lots of pent up pressure and stress by gently walking around like this.

As time went on though and healing began to take place, I found it difficult to maintain this newly found pleasure owing to pressures of work. I am sure, though, with discipline and good planning, it could become a regular feature in my life.

It would be wrong to suggest that my Christian belief is the only way forward. Not everyone has religious beliefs and if they do they may not be like my own. The book would not be complete without considering other methods by which people may want to cope with a bowel disorder that may or may not lead to surgery.

Some manage by being continuously positive. They have the attitude that a glass is half full rather than half empty. No matter what comes their way, such people are able to face things head on, showing very little emotion or weakness. Working with bereaved people I have been amazed by how a small proportion of people have the ability to project themselves through extremely painful times showing very little in the way of hurt or remorse. Somehow they have been able to get on with their lives living under extreme conditions.

Not all of us, however, are able to be so constantly positive in our attitudes, values and beliefs. There are practical techniques that can provide relief or comfort in which pain, stress, anxiety, fear, anger and other negative physical and mental conditions associated with disease can be alleviated. It should be emphasised, however, that the methods outlined below cannot cure anything; they can only alleviate some of the physical and mental symptoms associated with disease. It is suggested that the alternative therapies outlined below may be most helpful in helping sufferers to focus on living their daily lives with a bowel disorder and the lead up to, and aftermath, of stoma surgery.

If we were in a boat at sea in a raging storm and at risk of drowning, it would be helpful for our survival if we threw things overboard. This would help the boat to gain a better balance and ensure a better possibility of making it back to dry land. Similarly, there may be certain things that hold us back in our new lives as ostomists. We may have to shed things to survive. These may be either mental, such as ideas, or physical, in terms of possessions. We may have to make changes to meet new demands that have been enforced upon us. We may be able to meet these changes adequately, but then again we may have difficulty in doing this. A faith or general belief, even if it's simply believing in yourself, can be so helpful for survival.

As an ostomist, feeling good about yourself and having a good self-image is extremely important. If you've had surgery that leaves you with low self-esteem, it is extremely important that you begin to analyse and change your thinking so that you can find a way through. Bowel disorders can be very stressful. When they lead to surgery the stress is even greater as the operation is hard to come to terms with. The bottom can be knocked out of your life and emotions can begin to bubble. At this point it is very important to consider questions such as the following:

- What is important enough in my life to give it a meaning?
- In my present situation, what helps me to cope?
- Is there anything meaningful in my life or anything that especially frightens me at the moment?
- What could ease the worry, anxiety or pain?
- Am I at peace with myself?
- Do I need to explore this with someone who understands what I am going through?

You need to really think through these questions and provide answers to them. If in answering the questions you find that you need help to cope with your present life, where do you go for help, encouragement and to seek solace at a time like this? Perhaps some counselling or one of the alternative therapies listed below might help. Alternatively you might like to visit your GP for advice on how to manage.

In this chapter I first consider counselling and then look at a number of alternative therapies: the Alexander Technique, aromatherapy, meditation, yoga and bio feedback training. These provide different approaches to alleviating the side effects of bowel disease. You may find one or more than one of these techniques helpful.

Counselling

Counselling is a method of helping human beings with their difficulties. It can be extremely productive in helping people to overcome the major hurdles that they are facing at any given time. Rooted in psychotherapy, there is a focus on the one-to-one relationship, that is, counsellor and client, although group counselling is also prevalent. Clients are helped to reach decisions themselves without an opinion being offered by the counsellor. Clients may find this difficult at first but decisions can be successfully attained when a relationship of trust is achieved where clients realise that the counsellor cares about them. This is usually achieved by the counsellor using such skills as empathy, that is, learning to understand clients so well that their feelings, thoughts and motives are readily understood. Counsellors should also possess good attending skills. Here the counsellor shows his or her clients that they are really being listened to. The counsellor uses good eye contact and reflects back some of the conversation to the clients. Honesty, together with being willing to listen without interruption, can put the seal on a good professional relationship.

Today there are many opportunities for counselling. Individuals can have private counselling, where sessions may take place in the counsellor's office or arrangements can be made to visit at home. This, however, can be quite expensive and great care should be taken to ensure that the counsellor is fully qualified and accredited.

Most GP's surgeries have their own in-house counsellors, and your GP may be able to make a referral for you. There may well be a long waiting list, however, and the appointments may not be as regular as you might expect. The hospital or stoma nurse may be able to help regarding counselling. I suggest this might be the best way of obtaining a counsellor as it may lead to a more successful conclusion.

Whatever route you choose to take, it is most essential that you take care to select a counsellor who is fully qualified. An unqualified counsellor is not going to be able to help you in any way at all.

The initial session comprises an information-gathering process, where the counsellor encourages you to 'tell your story'. Through observational skills and careful listening, the counsellor will attempt to help you to find a way through your problem. The ultimate goal will be to help you to be able to face up to your situation without you needing any further help. Counselling helps to build up strength and confidence and promotes growth and empowerment of the client. It helps the client to take control of the given situation.

Counselling may well be able to help you to come to terms with the prospect of stoma surgery and living life with a stoma.

Further information from the British Association for Counselling and Psychotherapy (BACP), BACP House, 35-37 Albert Street, Rugby, Warwickshire CV21 2SG; 0780 440 5255.

The Alexander Technique

This technique was named after its creator, a Tasmanian, Frederick Matthias Alexander 1869 – 1955 who was a trained actor.

This is a very gentle technique of body alignment and release. The teacher guides the student or patient to lengthen and balance the body and encouragement is given to maintain this bodily poise and ease in everyday life. This is designed to improve posture and so avoid physical strain.

This technique may alleviate back pains, postural disorders, whiplash injury, breathing problems, myalgia, hypertension anxiety, stress and other chronic conditions. Again this technique may help to address the stress and anxiety that the Ostomist is under.

More information from The Society of Teachers of the Alexander Technique, 1st Floor, Linton House, 39-51 Highgate Road, London NW5 1RS; 0845 230 7828.

Aromatherapy

Aromatherapy is a method of treating bodily ailments with natural essential plant oils. This is usually in combination with a massage and inhalation. The oils are extracted from various herbs, flowers and trees. They may be used in small amounts during a massage, aromatic baths, inhalations and various cosmetic preparations. Trained aroma therapists believe in treating the whole person and used consistently, this technique has had a beneficial affect where more conventional ones have failed.

Aromatherapy, it is claimed, can be quite helpful in having a calming and analgesic effect on the person who is being treated. The majority of oils are highly antiseptic so are useful in the treatment of infections. Most essential oils have a specific effect on the emotional and physical level. I personally have witnessed the positive effect on terminally ill patients within the hospice where I work. As the vapours have been inhaled, they have provided a satisfying and relaxing effect.

Both Crohn's and Colitis sufferers have also benefited from receiving aromatherapy. Lemongrass and Neroli/Orange Blossom are claimed to be particularly successful in bringing relief as they address stress related conditions such as bowel disorders and provide a calming and relaxing effect together with having a stimulating effect on the whole system.

Further information from the Aromatherapy Consortium, P O Box 6522, Desborough, Kettering, Northamptonshire, NN14 2YX; 0870 7743477.

Meditation

Relaxation techniques are most effective in spells of mild or moderate anxiety. This can be achieved in a number of complementary techniques such as meditation. The conventional method involves slow breathing, muscle relaxation and mental imagery.

Meditation has been used in almost all major religions but is mostly linked to Buddhism and Hinduism. It offers a way in which the participant may be able to cope with the hectic pace of life and reconnect with a sense of who we really are. In this we may then gain control of our thoughts and feelings, finding a sense of peace and calmness that may help us deal with what life has dealt us.

This is yet another alternative that may be able to offer the Ostomist, Colitis or Crohn's sufferer, a way of coping and thus bringing a sense of meaning to what has happened to them.

Further information from: the School of Meditation, 158 Holland Park Avenue, London W11 4UH; 020 603 6116.

Yoga

Yoga is one of the six classic systems of Hindu philosophy distinguished from the others by the marvels of bodily control and the supposed magical powers ascribed to its devotees.

Yoga holds the doctrine that through the practice of certain disciplines, a person may achieve freedom from the limitations of the flesh, the delusions of sense and the pitfalls of thought. A person may then attain union with the object of knowledge. This union is apparently the only true way of knowing.

Yoga is a way of bringing awareness to the self through the body. There are many types of yoga. In the West we are more familiar with hatha yoga. This deals primarily with posture and breathing. Other forms focus more on the spirit and meditation offering calmness and relaxation that may offer help to the mind and body.

Further information from: the British School of Yoga, Stanhope Square, Holsworthy, Devon EX22 6DF; 0800 7319271; or Iyengar Yoga Institute, 223a Randolph Avenue, London W9 1NL; 020 7624 3080.

Biofeedback Training

Biofeedback training is very useful in showing patients that they are not relaxed. Some may have become so used to being anxious that they fail to recognise this. Biofeedback will address this lack of knowledge.

It involves feeding back to the patient a physiological measure that is abnormal in anxiety. These measures may include electrical resistance of the skin of the palm, heart rate, breathing pattern or muscle electromyography.

Research has shown in studies on Biofeedback that it has appeared to have an effect in lowering blood pressure in a number of people.

Anxiety certainly figures quite strongly in someone who is suffering from Colitis or Crohn's Disease. It also is very strong in someone who has just received stoma surgery. It can be argued that this technique may be advantageous in bringing relaxation to the anxious sufferer.

These are only a few suggestions and more justice would be given to each technique if a more thorough study was undertaken before making one's mind up. For myself, Christianity is the answer. It gives me the strength and encouragement to face each and every day. It is also not a remedy or a cure but a complete way of life. However, for others, any of the above may be the answer.

Whatever you decide is the best solution for helping you address anxiety, I urge you to give it all you have got. It can and will be most helpful and therapeutic in your new life as an ostomist. We all need something to lean on or aim for in life. Identify your method of help and go for it.

14

KEEPING FIT

Throughout this chapter I offer guidelines that might help ostomists follow a healthy and well-balanced diet. I also outline what I eat and drink, although in this connection it is important to remember that every individual is different, not only having his or her own likes and dislikes but also possible allergies to certain foods or other problems.

Many people think that an ostomist needs to follow a strict diet, but this is simply not true. Ostomists can eat and drink what they like, with certain limitations.

If you are an ostomist, it is important to chew your food well to help digestion and to avoid excessive wind and stomach cramps. Meals also need to be eaten at regular times and fairly often. Long gaps between meals can promote a build up of wind, which may cause excessive cramping pain within the gut. It may also lead to the pouch filling with air, which could cause a leak.

When you first have a stoma, it is best to eat little and often until you can build up to a more regular routine. I have found that it's helpful to eat at regular times rather than graze spasmodically, as eating this way helps to set the clock on the stoma. Even though the stoma works whenever it wants to and I have no control over it, nevertheless if I eat at regular times I can usually gauge when the bag will need emptying. This in turn allows a degree of freedom to go out and about.

Being relaxed really helps when you eat. Try to sit upright at a table instead of slouched on a settee. Making sure you sit at the table, eating your meal slowly and avoiding conversation can really help to digest the food.

Certain foods can cause diarrhoea. It is wise to try small amounts of these foods to begin with and then decide whether or not to include them as part of your diet. Such foods include highly spiced and fatty products, cabbage, beans, under-cooked vegetables, figs, prunes, bean sprouts, celery, lettuce and spinach. A large quantity of fresh fruit or pure fruit juices may also be unhelpful. You need a good balance of food to make sure that the consistency of the stool that ends up in the bag is not too watery, as it could be very embarrassing if it leaked out of the bag. If you do have diarrhoea it is most important you ensure that your fluid level is maintained. Otherwise you might become seriously dehydrated, which could be dangerous.

Whenever I have had a stomach upset and diarrhoea – and fortunately this is a rare event – my GP has prescribed codeine phosphate. (This prescription, however, may not be suitable for all ostomists.) On these occasions I have avoided spicy or fatty foods and dairy products, and have eaten dry toast until the stomach has returned to normal. I have also drunk a lot of non-alcoholic fluid to avoid dehydration.

If the output from the stoma is quite watery and there doesn't seem to be any apparent reason for this (such as a bug), I have eaten foods such as bananas, pasta, white rice or mashed potato to help thicken the output. It takes time to learn how to control what and how much you eat. Initially it may mean a number of phone calls to the stoma care nurses. I've found that they don't mind being contacted and have always been very helpful.

It is most important for an ostomist to drink plenty of fluid. You should drink a minimum of six to eight glasses of fluid a day to prevent dehydration, especially in hot weather. It is a good idea to carry a bottle of water around with you to meet this need.

Strenuous exercise will mean you will have to increase your daily intake of fluid. Holidays in hot climates or excessive sweating will also mean you will have to drink more. I often go out power walking or occasionally jog. I get very hot and usually sweat quite a lot when I do this. On these occasions I have to remind myself to take plenty of water.

Usually I eat and drink what I want, although I'm careful. The only foods that I've found difficult to eat are sweet corn and celery as I find them hard to digest. But I don't let eating any food worry me. If I find a particular food or drink that causes me a problem I leave it for a week or two and then try it again.

Alcohol affects ostomists just as much as it affects everyone else. Large quantities of beer or lager may result in loose stools. It may also cause excessive wind and may mean the bag will need emptying more than usual. Also it might be wise to bear in mind that having a stoma and drinking a great deal of alcohol might be a recipe for disaster.

The colostomist still has a colon so that most foods can be digested properly. The ileostomist on the other hand does not have a colon and therefore certain foods may well be difficult to process and may cause pain and obstruction. Experts recommend that ileostomists should avoid too much intake of foods such as nuts, beans, sweet corn, coconut, tomato skins, dried fruit, popcorn, mushrooms, stringy vegetables, onions and most uncooked vegetables.

If a blockage occurs, which may be the result of eating one or some of the above-mentioned foods, you will notice that either the motion of the bowel from the stoma has stopped or that the bag contains excessive amounts of watery output. You may also notice that the stoma changes in colour and size. If this change is significant and you begin to feel unwell with stomach pains, nausea and vomiting, you should contact a doctor as soon as possible. You may then have to have an emergency visit to a hospital where treatment will be provided to clear the blockage. If the blockage is very serious, this may mean a resectioning of the remaining bowel, which will entail the removal of the blocked part of the small bowel.

Although I am mindful of expert advice I do feel strongly that it is for ostomists themselves to try out as many foods as they wish. Perhaps trying a little of something rich and strange is better than never trying anything out of the ordinary.

I have found skins on fruit and vegetables difficult to digest. Thus, if I'm going to eat a salad, I tend to cut the skin off tomatoes and, with fruit, always peel apples and pears before eating them. I avoid eating segments of an orange as I find the skins on the segments difficult to digest.

As ileostomists don't have a colon they suffer a loss of salt as well as fluid. There is a need to increase the intake of salt to compensate for this. I find Marmite and Bovril useful for this, as well as packet or tinned soup. If, however, you suffer from high blood pressure or have diabetes you should consult your doctor about consuming any salty foods.

Foods that create a smell may be a problem. Fish, onions, cabbage, eggs, garlic, baked beans and asparagus may all cause an odour. But tomato juice, orange juice, yoghurt and parsley on the other hand may help to counteract this. If you want to, try odoriferous foods in small amounts at first and avoid them if you find they cause you too much embarrassment.

I consider myself to be a very clean person. I would be very upset if I found out that I smelt at all. It was bad enough when I had UC. I was continually checking myself to see if I smelt, or asking Hazel if she could smell anything. When I had the permanent ileostomy, I thought I would notice a quite distinct smell. How wrong I was. The only time that I've noticed any odour, apart from when the appliance is drained or changed, is when I've had a stomach bug. This is the same for everyone, whether or not an ostomist.

For the colostomist fibre is useful for keeping the bowel action regular. There is no nutritional value to be found in fibre, but it does absorb water. This in turn helps to add bulk to the food. Fibre may be useful in smaller quantities for the ileostomist. It can add enough bulk to ensure that the output is firm but soft enough to pass through the stoma safely. Fibre is found in cereals such as Shredded Wheat, Weetabix, muesli, wholemeal bread, pasta, rice, beans, and fruit and vegetables.

Fats are valuable for protecting vital organs of the body and for monitoring the body's temperature. There are two main types of fat: saturated and unsaturated. Saturated fats, such as those to be found in butter, meat, cheese and lard, tend to produce cholesterol, of which again there are two types, one 'good' and one 'bad'. Too much of the 'bad' cholesterol can lead to heart disease. Unsaturated fats on the other hand have very little effect on cholesterol, and some, such as vegetable oils like olive and sunflower oils, actually lower cholesterol levels. Many fish oils contain unsaturated fats, and a healthy diet should contain as much of these as possible as they have omega oils that can help prevent cardiovascular disease. We tend to eat too much fat, especially in fried foods. But it is wrong to say that all fats are bad for you; the body needs fats. It is best to eat foods that contain saturated fats in moderation.

If you want to increase your energy levels, you could increase your carbohydrate intake by consuming foods such as bread, pasta, potatoes, cereal and fresh fruit. But avoid sugary drinks and alcohol, cakes, chocolate, biscuits and sweets. It is essential that ostomists watch their weight. Being overweight can cause problems such as a retracted stoma where the stoma sinks into the abdominal wall. As yummy as sugary morsels are they are also, alas, counterproductive, as they tend to promote ill health. Also extra weight may cause leaks from the bag because the abdomen has increased in size.

I have found that dietary advice can be quite contradictory at times. It is confusing to be told to eat low fat foods but also to eat those that contain high fibre.

Increasingly, many restaurants and cafés use very little salt in cooking. For ileostomists this may be harmful, as they need to replace the salt lost as the result of the lack of a colon. If a salt cellar is available, this may be the answer. I, however, think that adding salt to unsalted cooked food never tastes the same as adding salt to food whilst it is being cooked.

If you are confused or unsure about what to eat, talk to your stoma care nurse who will certainly know about dietary matters.

When I first had my stoma I was paranoid about what to eat. Hazel and I talked a lot about foods I could and could not eat and sometimes had arguments about the subject of food. I initially lived in dread that I might eat the wrong thing, get an obstruction and be rushed into hospital. After a time, however, common sense began to prevail and I decided to eat some nice food. Little by little I began to experiment. A glass of wine here, a slice of pizza there, until I became confident enough to decide that I and no one else was going to choose what I was going to eat. It took a few weeks to take the plunge but I took it and now enjoy a good diet.

During the week I don't usually have breakfast. Some say I should but I never have and this works for me. (Breakfast is, however, thought to be a good idea.) At lunchtime, about 12.15, I have some sandwiches and a bag of low-fat crisps, followed with an apple and a banana. I then drink a cup of tea or coffee. I have my main meal in the evening, at about 6 p.m., perhaps later at about 7.30 at the weekends. This may consist of pasta or a chicken or ham salad. Occasionally I may have a steak with salad. But I choose not to eat a lot of red meat. Around about 9 p.m. I may have another bag of low-fat crisps or perhaps a banana and a drink, usually a fizzy one.

At weekends what I eat is different, but I still try to eat at the same times. On Saturdays we have a cooked breakfast, but as we have it around lunchtime it's really lunch. In the evening we might have some salad rolls, a pizza or the odd curry, together with a bottle of wine and/or some bottles of lager. We tend not to go out a lot – perhaps every six weeks or so – but when we do I'll usually drink lager. I limit this to no more than four pints in the whole evening. I suffer no ill effects from this and look forward to the treat.

Following a lot of research and stringent texts, the medical profession now thinks that probiotic foods may help to manage the remission of UC and Crohn's. Each of us has billions of bacteria living in the gut known as microflora. Probiotic foods contain live microbes that help to create a better mixture of bacteria within the intestine by increasing the numbers of 'friendly' bacteria that are able to survive through the stomach acid because they adhere to the intestine. Such foods are contained in yoghurts, fermented drinks and can be found in health food stores where they may be obtained in capsule and powder form, with names such as Acidophilus.

Tests on yoghurt are not yet conclusive, but research suggests that if you consume yoghurt you have a higher likelihood of being able to digest milk products, a quicker recovery from certain types of diarrhoea, enhanced immune function, reduction in certain cancers and possible lowering of blood cholesterol levels.

Because some of the 'friendly' bacteria have special nutrient requirements, it has been proposed that adding particular carbohydrate foods or nutrients known as prebiotics to the diet may be a way of increasing their number.

Prebiotic carbohydrates are found in certain types of fruit and vegetables. These include bananas, asparagus, garlic, wheat, tomatoes, Jerusalem artichokes, onions and chicory. The prebiotics are not digested but make their way to the gut where they enhance the 'friendly' bacteria by stimulating growth.

Researchers at the University of Dundee have developed a type of probiotic which, when combined with carbohydrates, forms a synbiotic. This has been shown to have a dramatic effect on UC sufferers, who on trials were found to have experienced reduced pain and a reduction in diarrhoea.

I am determined not to let my stoma rule me. I'm sensible and know my limitations, but I also want to live my life and enjoy it and so I do. I'm conscious about my weight and try to keep in good shape. At first this was impossible. Following the operation a small puff of wind would have blown me away with it. After a time, however, I began to eat more solids and the weight started to pile on. My weight was not helped by my large intake of chocolate. When I visited my surgeon for my first post-operative appointment he told me quite bluntly to lose some weight.

I'd noticed that my stomach had begun to get larger and that it was putting a strain on both my stoma and the bag. When I was first measured up for the stoma, just before the operation, I was much slimmer. As I didn't relish potential problems such as the flange leaking I decided to slim down.

I thought about some exercise. I considered jogging. At first this was short lived, because I only managed to get twenty yards down the road before I was exhausted. I decided it would be more sensible to begin slowly and began walking. I covered just under a mile until after a few months I began to get stronger. With dedicated walking and a sensible diet I managed to shed about half a stone. That was very satisfying. I then found I could jog without getting out of breath. I didn't push this too much, though, because at my age with a stoma I felt that what I was doing was enough.

I now try to exercise every night. This consists of quite vigorous walking, perhaps just less than two miles most evenings. It isn't possible all the time. But I've reached a level of fitness where I can miss the odd night. I'm not planning to join the next Olympics; I just want to keep fit and live life to the full.

15

LIFE IS WHAT YOU MAKE IT

When you have survived a potentially life-threatening major operation, not to mention the disease that pre-empted the surgery, it helps to see things in perspective. Following surgery and my convalescence I realised how important life is and how it can be taken away so quickly without warning.

At first it was difficult to get about, but after a few weeks I began to feel much stronger. I thought back to when I was in hospital and feeling so awful. Outside it had been windy and raining very heavily nearly all the time. Looking out of the window I could see people walking about, oblivious to the inclement conditions. I made a promise to myself that as soon as I got home and felt stronger I would also ignore the wind and the rain.

One day I decided to stand by my promise. Outside was terrible, but this didn't deter me. I put on wet weather gear, complete with Wellington boots, and much to the dog's surprise and panic and Hazel's displeasure I took the former out for a walk. The rain was teeming down but it didn't matter, except to the dog who got soaked. I was alive. I was out of hospital and healed, and I wanted to make the most of my freedom.

We walked into a wood and attempted to make it safely up a muddy track. As my Wellingtons didn't have a lot of grip I slipped over a couple of times. That, however, only led to the fun of it all. The stoma nurse would have been horrified, but I didn't care. I had my life back and wanted to fulfil the promise to myself. I was out for perhaps an hour before returning, slopping about all over the kitchen floor as I peeled off my wet garments one by one. The dog glared at me with distaste but it was my finest hour since returning home and I was overjoyed.

I began to realise that life has to be the greatest gift we possess, because without it we wouldn't possess anything. Jesus said something very interesting to His disciples about life, 'The thief does not come except to steal, and to kill, and to destroy. I have come that they may have life, and that they may have it more abundantly' (John 10:10). Jesus was obviously making a point here. As I studied His words I began to realise that the word abundantly in this context means an overflowing life that is filled with great and bountiful things. He wants to keep us well supplied and provided for in a lavish way, in other words, to live our lives to the full.

I also discovered that Jesus' intention is not only that we have life but also that we have it amazingly. He wants us to have it in total fullness, lacking nothing that is good for us: 'But those who seek the Lord shall not lack any good thing' (Psalm 34:10).

Yet it is so easy when things don't go the way we think they should to wish we had never been born, or, worse, to wish we were dead. I'm finding that there seems to be an in-built need for human beings to blame others when things go wrong. I myself have done this so many times. I have focused on the negative attributes of situations, feeling inadequate and sorry for myself, and have blamed other people for my misfortune. It shouldn't be like this.

I've discovered that life is for living and living to the full. It is the most valuable gift that could ever have been given to us and we need to hang on to it with all that we've got. I cannot describe how I felt when the test results showed there was no malignancy in my body. I had waited five days for the results and that time had seemed like years. It was a total relief when I heard the news. That incident has made me look long and hard at life. I now see how precious every moment of it is and that I need to make the most of every given opportunity.

Someone once said 'Life is what you make it'. I think to a certain extent that statement is true. We have to carve a way forward out of what we have. The choices we make today will determine what happens tomorrow. But the statement is not all that easy to accept. There are things forced on us that we could well do without such as sickness and death. We cannot make any provision for them; they just happen. Sometimes events that happen seem totally set against us and no matter what we do we don't seem to be able to find a way through.

I have found over the years that life can be very unpredictable. For instance, one minute I would feel that I was on top of UC. It would go into remission and there would be no sign of it returning. But suddenly it would return with a vengeance and the bottom would fall out of my world. I would sink into a pit of despair and I could well have done without this. At times like this it makes you feel like shouting 'It's not fair', because it definitely is not. At times it may seem that everyone else is doing well except you. I've also thought like this, but I know that compared to some people I have everything.

Almost a year after surgery I became a bereavement counsellor in a local hospice. I was completely humbled when I met the lovely people there. I was working with people who had been diagnosed with a terminal illness and who only had weeks to live. When people are facing death a counsellor will help the patient and/or family to face up to this. Some may be angry, in denial, or depressed. It may be possible, however, to help them reach a place of 'terminality', that is, the space in between the dying stage, which may be days, weeks or months away. At terminality people can be helped to face up to their situation, make the most of the time left and talk about things that may not have been said before to avoid regret or guilt at a later stage. It can be a very positive time, when the funeral is planned and the patient is helped to approach death with dignity, which in turn can help family and friends who are still living.

Most of these people and their families had very positive attitudes, even though their time for living was short. Although their emotions had been shattered, nevertheless they had decided that whatever time they had left they were going to live it to the full as best they could.

I have been working at the hospice now for five years and I'm amazed at the way people handle their situations. Although they struggle with the concept of dying and the lead up to it, and also struggle with the pressure and fear the idea of dying may be to them and their family and friends they are leaving behind, most approach their final moments with great dignity.

I realised that I too might have had cancer and might have ended my life in a hospice. Thankfully, however, I was spared and I am so grateful. When I'm tempted to think that life has dealt me a bad deal I remind myself where I've been and that I have life. It might not be what I would have chosen, but it's still life. How dare I not make the most of it?

We have to make the most of what we've got. We need to make a way where there doesn't seem to be one. This may seem to be impossible but I believe that it can be done. We have to forge a way forward to establish the ground, in other words, we have to keep thinking positively. It may then be easier to determine the way ahead.

When I had gone through surgery, I didn't really know what I would be doing next. I believed that God had shown me that He would use me, but I had no idea what for. I had qualifications. I had studied hard at university for them. But I had lost not only my job but my confidence as well. I couldn't see a way forward. Nevertheless there was one. I couldn't see it at first but it was there. Gradually the way opened up for me and now what I do is far better than what I did before. Also I am so much happier in doing what I do now in comparison to what I did before.

There is also a way for you. You may not see it right now, but allow a little time. Wait until you're healed and feel a little stronger, and the way may be there to take you on a little further. There is life after stoma surgery. It is not the end, even though you may feel it is at first. Look for the way. Reach out to your faith, or, if you are not a believer, at least have faith in yourself. Whatever you do don't give up.

That is the way it's been for me. I believe that God has made a way for me where there was not one before. Over the years He has got me out of so many scrapes and times of great injustice. When I've not been able to find a solution He has been there with His guiding hand and help.

Nevertheless I've still had to suffer. I had to go through ten years of suffering with UC and then have surgery. I could well have done without that time, but that was my life and I had to put up with it.

It is so easy to take things for granted. We can be so selfish at times that all we see is the 'I' in our lives. I have marked off a section in my Bible and written, 'Watch the "I" and "Me" in your life'. This is concentrated around verses in Philippians: 'Let nothing be done through selfish ambition or conceit, but in lowliness of mind let each esteem others better than himself. Let each of you look out not only for his own interests, but also for the interests of others.' (Philippians 2:3-4).

It is so easy in this day and age to concentrate only on oneself. We live in a world that is full of pressure and attempting to keep up with the pace of the material world often means we become self-centred, greedy and ungrateful. I hang my head in shame at the times I have called upon God to help me and when He has, marvellously, I have not thanked Him or been grateful.

How many times do we Christians enter into prayer with our 'I want this' and 'Please help me'? How wonderful it would be to come into God's presence and just thank and praise Him for who He is. But the world teaches us to be competitive and grab all we can, and sometimes that is all I have done.

If I have learnt one thing from the operation, it is to be thankful. I am so thankful to Hazel for her constant love, care and support. I am so thankful to the nurses and doctors who used their skill and expertise to get me to where I am now. Further thanks go to my family for their love and support. I am so thankful to the many people who sent me get-well cards and prayed for me to get better. Also I'm grateful to the people who visited me. And I'm totally thankful to my Heavenly Father who I believe brought all of this about. I would not have survived without Him, that is for sure. He made a way when there seemed to be no way.

I believe that God loved me enough to be with me when I was in hospital to bring me through the ordeal. What I've experienced has made me ask myself if I've fully realised how much He really loves and cares for His children. Psalm 120:1 says 'In my distress I cried to the Lord, and He heard me.' He was not too busy. I didn't have to book an appointment. He heard His child call and rushed to my aid.

Since I became a Christian in 1980 I have felt the call of God on my life for various commissions. My main commission from Him, however, is to let people know what He has to offer the world (Matthew 28:18-20). I believe that God wanted me to write this book and through it demonstrate His love to whoever reads it. I also believe He wants me to reach out to the many people who are suffering in one form or other from a bowel disorder and who have or will be undergoing surgery.

'Life is what you make it' means that you can create life out of what is given to you. You can, it is hoped, benefit from whatever you put into your life. The outcome may be different to what is intended, but if you don't make an effort to press forward and make something of the situation you are in you will get nowhere. It is up to you.

The African impala is an agile little creature. Whenever it is cornered by, for instance, a leopard or lion it can jump about twelve feet in the air and cover a space of about thirty feet. But if the impala were placed in a four-foot high walled enclosure, not chained but free to move, it wouldn't move. It would stay still trapped in fear. It wouldn't be able to see over the wall and would thus not be able to see the way ahead, so it would remain static.

Don't be like this. You may not be able to see the way forward right now. But be assured that there is one and that it is positive. Relax and give yourself time. You will get there.

To conclude, I love the following verse: 'And we know that all things work together for good to those who love God, to those who are the called according to His purpose.' (Romans 8:28). As a Christian I know that in bad times, when I'm treated wrongly or when bad things happen and disappointment prevails, God is in the situation with me and will help me through it successfully. He may not change things. The situation may remain the same or even get worse, but I believe that ultimately He promises that he will bring me through the bad times, thus adding to my maturity and character.

There is a lot of living to do and you can make a difference to someone's life by allowing him or her to see how you handle a situation positively. Wearing a bag may not be what you had planned for your life, nevertheless it is for life and you need to make the most of it. Stoma nurses are looking for volunteers who have been through stoma operations and who would be willing to talk to people who are waiting for the same operation. You could talk to these people. You are experienced because you have been through the operation and know what you are talking about. Make the most of this opportunity and help someone in need, like you were. You will most certainly make a difference to someone's life.

USEFUL INFORMATION

AMCARE (ConvaTec)
Order Line 0800 88 50 50
ConvaTec Free Customer Help Line 0800 282 254
email amcare.order@bms.com

British Colostomy Association
15 Station Road, Reading, Berks RG1 1LG
0118 939 1537/ Helpline 0800 328 4257
See Website for Membership details, Booklets and Support Groups
email sue@bcass.org.uk   Website www.bcass.org.uk

Continence Foundation
For people with bladder and bowel problems
Tel 01536 533255
email info@bladderandbowelfoundation.org
Website www.continence-foundation.org.uk

ConvaTec UK
Leaders in stoma care
Stoma care 0800 282 254
Wound care 0800 289 738
Website www.convatec.co.uk

Digestive Disorders Foundation
The charity for research and information on digestive disorders
PO Box 251, Edgware, Middlesex, HA8 6HG; 020 7486 0341
email ddf@digestivedisorders.org.uk
Website www.digestivedsorders.org.uk

Grahame and Hazel Howard's Support and Carer's Advice
email g.howard455@btinternet.com

Ileostomy and Internal Pouch Support group (ia)
National Office, Peverill House, 1-5 Mill Road, Ballyclare, Co.
Antrim, BT39 9DR; 0800 0184 724 / 028 9334 4043
See the website for membership details, booklets and support groups
email info@iasupport.org   Website www.the-ia.org.uk

National Association for Colitis and Crohn's Disease (NACC)
4 Beaumont House, Sutton Road, St Albans, Herts. AL1 5HH
See the website for membership details, booklets and local support groups;
0845 130 2233 email nacc@nacc.org.uk Web Site www.nacc.org.uk

National Key Scheme
To gain entry into disabled toilets
Radar, 12 City Forum, 250 City Road, London, EC1V 8AF;
Tel. 020 7250 3222
email radar@radar.org.uk Website www.radar.org.uk
Ring for prices for key
The NKS Guide: Accessible Toilets for Disabled People
(over 6000 toilets)

Stomacare
Support and advice for people with a stoma or bowel disorders
www.stomacare.org.uk

White Rose Collection Ltd
For underwear and products for people with stomas, from people with stomas
PO Box 5121, Wimborne, Dorset BH21 7WG;
01202 854634 email info@WhiteRoseCollection.com
Website www.whiterosecollection.com

Recommended Reading

Peter Cartwright, *Probiotics for Crohn's and Colitis*, Prentice Publishing, PO Box, 1704, Ilford, IG5 0WN, 2003

Peter Cartwright, *Coping Successfully with Ulcerative Colitis*, Sheldon Press, 2004

Dr Craig White, *Living with a Stoma*, Sheldon Press, 1997

Dr Craig White, *Positive Options for Living with your Ostomy*, Hunterhouse 2002

(Both these two latter books are available on email drcawhite@aol.com)